The International Library of Psychology

CONVERSATIONS WITH CHILDREN

T0174024

Founded by C. K. Ogden

The International Library of Psychology

DEVELOPMENTAL PSYCHOLOGY
In 32 Volumes

CONVERSATIONS WITH CHILDREN

DAVID KATZ AND ROSA KATZ

First published in 1936 by
Routledge, Trench, Trubner & Co., Ltd.

Reprinted in 1999 by
Routledge
2 Park Square, Milton Park, Abingdon, Oxfordshire OX14 4RN
711 Third Avenue, New York, NY 10017
First issued in paperback 2014

Routledge is an imprint of the Taylor and Francis Group, an informa company

Transferred to Digital Printing 2007

© 1936 David Katz & Rosa Katz
Translated from the German By Herbert S Jackson

The publishers have made every effort to contact authors/copyright holders
of the works reprinted in the *International Library of Psychology*.
This has not been possible in every case, however, and we would
welcome correspondence from those individuals/companies
we have been unable to trace.

These reprints are taken from original copies of each book. In many cases
the condition of these originals is not perfect. The publisher has gone to
great lengths to ensure the quality of these reprints, but wishes to point
out that certain characteristics of the original copies will, of necessity, be
apparent in reprints thereof.

British Library Cataloguing in Publication Data
A CIP catalogue record for this book
is available from the British Library

Conversations with Children
ISBN 978-0-415-20992-2 (hbk)
ISBN 978-0-415-75795-9 (pbk)

Developmental Psychology: 32 Volumes
ISBN 978-0-415-21128-4
The International Library of Psychology: 204 Volumes
ISBN 978-0-415-19132-6

To

PROFESSOR SAMUEL ALEXANDER

CONTENTS

PREFACE TO ENGLISH EDITION

In view of the strong interest with which the development of child psychology is watched in all English speaking countries, no special justification is needed for the English edition of a book which tries to apply an entirely new method to the problems of this branch of psychology.

The English edition of our book differs from the German one in so far as it brings a report of only 141 conversations instead of 154. The thirteen talks which have been left out have the character of " confessional talks ". The purpose of those confessional talks was to give the children an opportunity to get rid of a pressure from which they might suffer for a small offence they had committed. We hold now, as ever, that this category of conversations can have an excellent effect on children, but some people have raised objections to them. They maintain that the generalization of the method and its application by parents or teachers without the necessary psychological delicacy might do more harm than good.

We feel very much indebted to Mrs. Susan Isaacs for the deep interest she has taken in the translation of our book.

We are particularly grateful to our friend Mr. Herbert S. Jackson for undertaking the tedious and time-consuming task of translation.

PREFACE

About two years ago we began from purely private motives to note down word for word conversations which we had carried on with our children. What parents who have had the privilege of enjoying the refreshing intercourse with the unfolding mind of a child would not have cherished the desire to capture as many of their utterances as possible and to record them in a permanent form, so that their refreshing flavour might be used again and again in later years to sweeten the stale affairs of humdrum everyday life ? Time hurries on, the years of naturalness are soon over, and as soon as he goes to school the child becomes ever more firmly entangled in the tragedy of civilization, and his expressions lose much of the delightful charm of originality. Many of the most characteristic expressions can be captured in the ordinary photograph, and still more by film and sound recording. Systematic collecting can gather together sketches, plastic work, and handwork of all kinds in which the child's creative forces were developed and fixed. We did not omit to use any of these means in our desire to create the most effective means of helping us to remember the children in the various stages of their development. But we soon discovered that nothing is capable of reflecting their personality so directly as dialogues taken down word for word, which were carried on with them on all kinds of occasions. The conversations were therefore to be aids to our memory, and as such they were taken down in our note-books. But when we realized in course of time what unusually rich material for investigation into child-psychology was contained in them, we determined to publish them, not without a certain inner conflict, which will be readily understood from the intimate nature of the material.

The fact that many of the children's utterances are reminiscent of those expressions found in periodicals under such headings as " These Children ", might lead some readers to a false interpretation of the aim of our work, and cause them to assume that we are more concerned with affording amusement than instruction. Such a conception would entirely miss the strictly scientific aim we had in view in publishing the conversations. That the material yielded by the children is amusing at times ought not in itself to be any obstacle to its utilization in the most serious scientific investigations.

In the present volume we shall analyse 141 conversations. All statements made here refer to the state of affairs up to the date of the last recorded conversation. In the meantime the children's development has undergone many important changes, which could scarcely have been foreseen. The reception accorded to this present volume will determine whether we shall report on these developments by means of a further selection from the already numerous conversations we have since recorded.

Would it not have been sufficient to publish a smaller number of dialogues? We believe that the broad base of numerous conversations is necessary in order to obtain clear outlines of the form and content of the world of the child. Moreover, in these conversations we have aimed at providing a collection of material for other child psychologists, and as such it can never be extensive enough to supply all the varied requirements of those utilizing it.

The more abundant the material, the greater is the probability that every one will discover something for his purpose, whatever his interest may be—the child's imagination, his thinking, his feelings, his wish-pictures—whether it be the form or the content of the world of the child, there will be something for him. In any case even those who cannot subscribe to our interpretations of the conversations will at least find in them valuable raw material.

DAVID KATZ,
ROSA KATZ.

INTRODUCTION

Purpose and General Point of View of the Investigation

Conversations which we have had with our children form the main content of the present work. Whatever may be the attitude adopted towards our attempted analysis of the dialogues as regards content and form, and towards the general conclusions for child-psychology and pedagogy which we have considered ourselves justified in drawing, the conversations themselves will always be able to claim a certain value in themselves as a source of material for investigation into child-psychology—a source which at present stands alone in the whole literature of child psychology. The very fact that it will later on be possible to determine how children in a family spoke and were spoken to at this definite time, would justify the recording of such conversations. The history of pedagogy gives us instances of artificially constructed (didactic) conversations,[1] but the actual dialogue of conversations with children reported word for word would have been of much more value for our understanding of the position of the child in the family and in society.

We were impelled to the publication of these dialogues chiefly by theoretical motives—we desired thereby to make a contribution to pure research. But the investigation also yields material of considerable value to pedagogy. The conversations did not originate in the psychological laboratory ; the vast majority of them were derived from natural everyday intercourse with our children, and what conversation carried on with one's child is devoid of educational influences, whether one intends them or not ? Many

[1] In this connection we may mention the fictitious conversations in Salzmann's *Krebsbüchlein*.

conversations are however of a definitely pedagogical nature. Together with the consideration of the question of the awakening of conscience, they make up the main subject-matter of the section in which the considered pedagogical conclusions are set forth.

In the literature of child psychology there are available standard investigations into the way in which a child masters the language of his environment up to the point where the technical acquisition of language may be considered complete, but Stern [1]—and it is to him and his wife that we owe the most thorough monograph on the development of the language of the child—has himself pointed out that quite new problems arise if we consider the speech of the child as a connected expression of his personal life and experience. Here, too, atomistic methods of consideration have usually overlooked the natural totalitarian starting point, which is, of course, conversation. We certainly do meet in treatises by competent authorities isolated reports of shorter or longer conversations carried on by children amongst themselves or with adults, but it is soon discovered that these conversations are quoted as documents of *individual* childish thinking, desiring, and feeling, and that the point of view of social psychology has been entirely neglected in favour of this individual standpoint. To the Swiss psychologist Piaget must go the credit for having made this point of view (i.e. the progress of the socialization of thought in children's conversation) the starting point of a programme of investigation.[2] Piaget's work is chiefly concerned with conversations carried on by children amongst themselves during play or other occupation. The dialogues in which adults took part are less numerous and these latter again are predominantly not informal but guided and directed towards a definite goal

[1] Stern, W., *Psychologie der frühen Kindheit*, 4 ed., p. 146, Leipzig, 1927 (quoted as Stern).

[2] Piaget, J., (a) *Le langage et la pensée chez l'enfant*, Neuchatel et Paris, 1923 (quoted as Piaget I) ; (b) *Le jugement et le raisonnement chez l'enfant*, Neuchatel et Paris, 1924 (quoted as Piaget II).

and are therefore more in the nature of test conversations (Piaget II, p. 179 ff.). Our conversations are, on the contrary : (1) Almost without exception, conversations between children and adults ; (2) Almost exclusively informal, spontaneous conversations. Both of these facts have contributed to produce essential differences in the structure of these conversations. Piaget discovered that the conversation of younger children does not always reveal a true connection between statement and counter-statement : he states that we get rather the expression in monologue of individual feeling and thoughts, or we get statements which, even though occasioned by the presence of this or that person, yet are not intended to call forth any verbal response. In his view speech obtains its full social function only in later childhood ; but even in the case of a 5 year old child he computes the number of egocentric statements to be as high as 50 per cent of all recorded expressions. With reference to these statements by Piaget, Stern remarks : " It is certain that we have here a difference between the language of early childhood and that of the adult, a difference which has its origins deep in the totally different personal structure of the child " (Stern, p. 147). But Stern is quite right in pointing out that the unusually high percentage of egocentric statements in Piaget's results is probably due to the special social conditions in the Children's Home at Geneva, where the observations were carried out. And in a test of Piaget's findings at a Kindergarten in Hamburg, where the children formed a somewhat closer social group, Martha Muchow discovered little more than a third of the remarks of 5 year old children to be egocentric.[1] So when we have the more intimate contact of children living amongst family influences we are justified in expecting a still greater reduction in the percentage of egocentric remarks. The child's courage in social conversation, and his possibility of replying to the statements of others must of course grow

[1] Muchow, M., *Das Montessori-System und die Erziehungsgedanken Friedrich Fröbels*, Leipzig, 1926.

in proportion as his own means of expression and capacity to make himself understood become increasingly similar to those of others and in proportion as his world of ideas and philosophy of life (Weltanschauung) become increasingly similar to those of his environment. The most favourable conditions for this development are provided in the family. Our observations showed that the remarks of our two children, even from the time when the younger of them was only 3 years old, were not predominantly egocentric when they were playing with each other. But if at the same period they were with strange or less familiar children, then their way of expression changed in the direction of increased egocentricity.[1] We find therefore that in their conversation children either do not understand or do so less readily than adults. This is connected not only with the original higher egocentricity, but also with other circumstances. Children who grow up in different environments must experience the difficulty of making social contact through speech in the same way as adults who speak different languages. It is of course obvious that the level of conversation of children amongst themselves will always be lower than that between children and adults. We would even go so far as to assert that the utterances of a child in the presence of its parents are only in the rarest cases egocentric. This applies even to children in the stage of one word sentences with their emotional volitional character, and so it is true to a still greater extent of the children whose dialogues are to be reported here.

What has been our aim in these investigations? We wished to determine what the child does with his language, after he has learned in some measure to use technically this magic key which unlocks all the doors of higher knowledge. How does the child's dialectic develop? With the acquisition of speech the child begins for the first time to be a real human being. However important for the

[1] Investigations into intimacy and distance in social relationships could be carried out in the nursery, just as W. Stok has undertaken them for adults. *Zeitschrift für angerwandte Psychologie*, 28, 1927.

child's maturing his personal contact with things may be, instruction has a much greater effect. The acquisition of the traditional cultural values takes place by means of question and answer, assertion and counter-statement in innumerable varying forms of discussion.[1] What are the phases in the development of dialogue? We shall attempt to discover them for a period of several years by means of the analysis of conversations carried on with our children. We may mention at once that there still remains the task of carrying on these investigations when the children are of school age, and indeed beyond that up to the years of maturity and to the debates which take place between adults on any intellectual topic. The phases in the development of dialogue are extremely illuminating for the " Lebensform " of the child. The content of the conversations serves as a criterion for the thinking, feeling, and volitional attitudes taken up by the child towards his environment in general; it determines principally what we may designate as the world of the child. However important a child's sense perception, actions (either playful or serious), and manual creations may be for the interpretation of his world, nothing is so revealing for this purpose as his verbal utterances when he begins to have some command of language. In some way or another everything forces its way eventually into verbal expression. Thus our conversations also are to be of assistance in sketching the world of the child. If we at first obtain individual, childish images (Weltbilder) we shall have to test to what degree they are to be accepted as typical.[2]

[1] The greater emphasis laid on social-psychological points of view will probably lead us to interpret many things in the history of the evolution of speech in a different way from formerly. An individual psychological standpoint is for instance revealed by H. Gutzmann, " Psychologie der Sprache ", *Kafka's Handbuch der vergleichenden Psychologie*, vol. 2, Munich, 1922, " Speech as a movement of expression is at first merely a way of releasing and discharging inner tension. It is of secondary importance as a means of communicating inner processes."

[2] Piaget has also dealt with the portrayal of the childish image (Weltbild), *La représentation du monde chez l'enfant*. Paris, 1926.

We shall most accurately characterize the majority of the conversations reported here if we designate them as " chats ". We never spoke to our children in a formal, superior style, but endeavoured to keep the conversation as simple and natural as the circumstances permitted. Our instruction was never done forcibly. Our answers to the children's question's or the questions that we deemed it necessary to ask were adapted as far as possible to each individual situation. With a clear conscience we can state that thoughts of producing a striking effect for publication have never misled us into guiding the process of conversation otherwise than as mentioned above. The more so, as the idea of publishing the conversations only occurred to us several months after we had begun to record them for our personal use. But even after we had resolved to publish the conversations, we allowed no change to take place in our method of carrying on the dialogues, nor have we tried to create a sensation by selecting from amongst the recorded conversations a number of dialogues with particularly witty or precocious remarks in the children's answers. Our endeavour has been to convey the intellectual level through the ordinary average conversations of the children so that they may appear neither cleverer nor duller than they really are. We have tried to present impartial accounts of the two children, both from the point of view of ability and also of character. In portraying the personalities of our children we have therefore endeavoured to proceed *sine ira et studio*. But if anyone feels inclined to think that the natural urge of parents to idealize their own children must be taken into account even with parents who are psychologists, let him make for himself any correction which he deems necessary. Should it even be true, as he may consider, that we have tended to suppress or censor those conversations with a downright foolish or immoral character, even that would in no wise lessen the value of the conversations actually reported, in so far as they are striking for their high level. More than once we were struck by remarks of the children which seemed to us extraordinary performances, totally incredible in children of their age ; but similar flashes of genius are reported by almost all careful observers of children of pre-school age. The younger child displays occasionally an insight bordering on genius— but one must be on one's guard against giving it an intellectualistic interpretation. Not without good reason did Goethe speak of a period of genius in the life of every human being.[1]

The conversations which took place were previously designated positively as " chats ", and the term was used in order to indicate that they were kept free from everything savouring of instruction, work, or tests. The only exceptions are a few dialogues whose " experimental " nature will be obvious save when mention is made of our purpose. The relation of the informal chat to the conversation with an ulterior motive is the same as that of play to work. At play the child, so long as he is not restricted by rules, acts quite free from any compulsion. In just the same way we attempted in the majority of our conversations to keep clear of anything which might have been felt as compulsion. This was best achieved—negatively—when we set ourselves no problem to be solved or goal to be reached in the conversation at issue. Every didactic conversation, even if it is to be a triumph of Socratic midwifery, has a definite goal, towards which the teacher directs it. The teacher never loses sight of this goal, however delicate the suggestions used may be, and even though he may have at times to interrupt his obstetric services because the idea to be worked upon does not yet seem to him ready for birth. In our chats as a rule the children fixed the various goals themselves. We

---

[1] " If children grew up according to early indications then we should have nothing but geniuses. But growth is not merely development ; the various organic systems which go to the making of one man originate one from another, follow each other, change into each other and even consume each other, so that after a certain time scarcely a trace is to be found of many of these capacities and manifestations of power." *Dichtung und Wahrheit.*

helped them to reach these goals, as long as their inclination tended along those lines, but if one goal replaced another, then we followed the new track. The conception of work is always to some degree connected with a goal exerting its influence from outside: in experience this corresponds to that consciousness of a task, the strain of which can be largely alleviated, but never entirely removed, even by the skilled pedagogue. It is easy for anyone knowing the child to recognize the manifestation of " task consciousness " in gesture and speech starting from the phonetics, the tone of voice, and proceeding to the last nuances in the construction of the whole sentence which makes up the answer.

The changes from didactic conversation to actual chatting are, of course, fluid, but we cannot consider as spontaneous even those conversations with a child which are begun in a simple testing process (this simplicity is of course to allay the excitement which has been previously caused by the consciousness of an examination) in order to induce a definite performance or perhaps merely to demonstrate that such a performance is impossible. Not only did we allow the conversations to proceed as spontaneously as possible, but even the starting point of many of the conversations can be designated as natural, in the sense that they had their origin in a question of one of the children, or if not in a question at least in an " interrogative assertion ", as we call that type of sentence which in its external form is a statement, but in its inner structure a question.[1] The answer given by us, or—when we were dealing with a " feeler " put forth by the child—the correction provoked, was always kept as close as possible to the information sought by the child in the case at issue. The child might

---

[1] The process of asking an assertion is met with amongst young people and even adults in cases where the person concerned is desirous either of avoiding committing an error or feels that a direct question would betray too much respect. Then the tendency is to *assert*, in the hope of provoking thereby the desired response. The experienced judge of character can tell at once from the rhythm of the sentence what is taking place.

either be satisfied by our reply, or feel itself impelled to ask a further question or make another assertion. In this way the conversation developed, till it somehow or other found a satisfactory conclusion. The impulse to give a new turn to the conversation or to choose a new topic was as a rule left entirely to the child. All this of course did not prevent us from exerting quite a decisive influence on the course of the conversations.

The second part of our work has as its object an examination, in the light of various conversations, of the effect upon the course of these conversations of the various answers given to the children by means of the question they were asked, and of the objections, corrections, additions, and replies of various kinds they received. Here we shall attempt briefly to characterize the general effect of the adult on the child expressing itself in speech. Differing from Piaget's statement we previously pointed out that the conversations which took place between our two children when playing together had a by no means predominantly egocentric character. But it is certain that the inclination to begin a dialogue was very much less when the two children were by themselves in the room or at least when they believed that they were alone, than when they were with their parents or with some other adult member of the household. It is also a proved fact that the dialogues which did actually take place between the two children were extremely low in quality and limited in range. In order to get a conversation started it is necessary to release a certain tension existing between person and person; a tension which can be proved as an actual psychical reality in experience. The origin of a psychical potential which is discharged in conversation depends on a great many influences, one of which is the age of the persons concerned. Even when the above-mentioned conditions for the possibility of mutual understanding are fulfilled, young children exert psychologically only a slightly inductive influence on each other. They expect little information from each other in conversation, and therefore do not seek it with any particular persistence. On the other hand every adult is at once felt by the child to be simply the adult who is superior, the authority who can aid him in every intellectual emergency. This applies also to adults who are complete strangers, in whose presence the child may remain completely silent through shyness. It may be that this relationship between child and adult is determined to some degree instinctively but certainly the decisive factor is the child's experience, so frequently repeated in the family-circle, that the adult is able to give answers to his questions. But in order to avoid any confusion at this point in our portrayal of the relationship, we shall first of all consider only the effect of well-known adults upon the child's readiness to speak, that is of members of the family and household. Even the silent presence of adults is enough to produce in a child a peculiar *attitude* which is revealed by his utterances. It is perfectly clear that he recognizes that he is no longer alone with his problems : he has only to ask the adult to find the way to their solution. But perhaps one should not choose this general formulation, but rather a more specialized one, in order to characterize the given social psychological state of affairs. The child is perfectly able to distinguish between the various adult members of the household and turns correspondingly to each of them with requests differing in each case. He can come to his father about things quite different from those for which he approaches his mother, to his parents again for things not to be brought to his grandmother, and she in turn stands closer to him than does his nursemaid. Accordingly conversations of quite different form and content develop with the various members of the household. It can be said with certainty that the child reveals a fresh mental level every time there is a change of conversation-partner. Indeed it is no exaggeration to maintain that the whole personality of the child seems to vary from one conversation-partner to another. From the starting-point of child psychology we are here making a modest beginning in the investigation of those questions of social psychology which concern the effect, one upon the other, of personalities in conversation. It is well known to what a high degree the starting of a conversation between any given persons depends on the mutual harmony of the characters : it is perhaps even more important than intelligence, education, or class level, all of which play such a decisive part in the sociological sphere. This applies also in the case of children, so that the same child may reveal marked variations in its readiness to talk to different members of its accustomed environment.

The adult will not always be able to understand the child's conversation in the way that he desires it to be understood, and the child will never understand the adult unless he tries to make himself intelligible. Thus there often arises a situation where each is talking past the other, and instead of a properly connected dialogue we get what Piaget terms a " collective monologue ". It has happened more than once in our experience with our own children that we were unable in any way to discover what their utterances meant, even though we certainly knew our children extremely well and although there was no person they knew so well as their mother. Many of the needs expressed in speech concern events about which the child alone knows ; others are intelligible only against the background of events that have indeed taken place in the family, but have made an impression only on the child, and accordingly have been remembered by him only. Every utterance of the child therefore and every conversation is to a large degree bound up with his whole past life. Every conversation of the child is coloured not only by his individual experience but also by his character, and this must be taken into account if the whole of the meaning is to be extracted from the conversation. This statement will be proved by numerous examples. Our last remarks demonstrate that it is only in the family of a child psychologist, and even there only in the most intimate contact with the children, that a really exhaustive analysis of children's conversations can be carried out.

How does one set about understanding the verbal utterances of a child ? Here we come to a special case of the general problem of understanding a child through its expressive behaviour, a case in which the various types of empathy become important. Elsa Köhler distinguishes between non-determining empathy (the intuitive understanding of a child's experience resulting involuntarily and occasioned by a spontaneous resonance in one's own ego) and determining empathy, by which is implied a voluntary placing of oneself in the child's position. The longer one lives with children and the more intimate one becomes with them, the more dominant becomes the non-determining type of empathy. It can lead to an astonishingly high degree of harmony with the psychical life of the child. As an example we may mention that one of us felt for a time that he was going through his childhood experiences again in our elder boy.[1] It is therefore not surprising that in these circumstances one can often predict quite accurately the behaviour of the child in some definite situation. The individual conversations themselves will give the clearest idea of how the child's understanding was shaped by his verbal utterances.

We stated above that every conversation with a child is coloured by his character and that its sense can only be fully grasped by taking into account the character behind it. The converse also applies, that nothing affords so deep an insight into children's characters as our method of free conversation. This would perhaps not have struck us so forcibly had not nature endowed the two children with quite different temperaments. Even if the conversations

---

[1] The following remarks from our scientific records are worthy of note in connection with the above. When the children were still being fed by their mother with soft food, she used to open her mouth almost convulsively at each spoonful she gave the child, just as the child did, or ought to have done. It was almost impossible for the mother to keep her mouth closed. Perhaps in addition to the non-determining empathy the opening of the mouth was also produced by the wish that the child should open its mouth wide in order not to hinder the feeding.

were to be given in fragments, these fragments would be quite sufficient to reveal the character of the speaker on each occasion. As far as we know, the science of human character study, which is now reviving, has not as yet concerned itself at all with tracing the development of character in children. Probably there is material bearing on this problem in the publications of psychoanalysts and of individual psychologists of Adler's school, but the obtaining of the psychological data suffers (owing to the specialized standpoints of these schools) from the prejudices of their individual points of view. In the second part of this work we shall sketch the characters of our two children in rather more detail, and we shall utilize not only the contents of the conversations themselves but also other notes from our scientific records.

The available literature of child psychology is rich in isolated verbal utterances of children in the form of shorter or longer sentences called forth by some occasion or other, but it is not always clear whether we have a spontaneous utterance, caused by the situation itself, or whether it is one caused in the first place by some other sentence. This may be of decisive importance for an estimation of the performance of the child in the realm of thought. A single sentence spoken by a child *may* be a unity in itself, but if it stands in the middle of some fairly long conversation it is so no longer. For then the higher sense-unit, superior to the individual sentence, is the whole dialogue that is carried on with the child ; in it are included as constructive elements all the utterances of all the persons concerned in the conversation up to its conclusion. A dialogue possesses an extremely peculiar structure. It is a complex development in time, produced by those taking part in it yet to some extent lying between them. The individual thinker in his study has complete freedom of movement in his deliberations, but in a dialogue or in a discussion with another person he must of necessity give up a part of that freedom. If he fails to do this and does not trouble to attend to what the other person is saying, then he is only uttering aloud his own self-determined independent thought. A person who listens to a dialogue without taking part himself judges the various links in the chain of the conversation according to their value and sense from the standpoint of the whole of the conversation. Thus the value of the individual links must remain, so to speak, unestimated, even when the conversation takes its normal course with no surprising turns.[1] Yet it is not only those not taking part, but chiefly the participants in the conversation who experience this structure-form of the dialogue. Those taking part in the discussion allow their later remarks to be influenced by previous ones, both their own and other people's : they experience the shifting of emphasis in the earlier parts of the conversation as it progresses, and finally look back on the whole as a unity, just as one looks back on a sonata as a unified piece of music when the last note has been played. The conditions in the dialogues in which children participate are fundamentally the same as those that we have just described. From this it is obviously necessary to investigate the conscious attitudes of children engaged in dialogues, for this field has up to the present been neglected by child-psychologists. It was bound to be neglected as long as the dialogue between child and adult was not regarded as a problem at all. The dialogue is the most natural and probably the most important form of the child's thought-development. Therefore, illuminating as the older methods of investigation of the child's thinking were in many respects, they were bound to overlook much that is immediately obvious to the newer methods of approach.

Many of the conversations recorded are governed by their situation. Of this type are those which are begun by the child because of his position at a certain moment, either playing or otherwise occupied. We find less frequently

---

[1] This remaining in suspense of individual links is also familiar to us from other sense units developing in time. (Novel, drama, film.)

conversations which are bound to some external situation. These we understand as conversations which in their development remain bound to the external situation or vary as the situation itself varies. By the side of these dialogues governed by the situation, or bound to it, we meet much more frequently spontaneous conversations, that is, those begun by the child himself without any external stimulus being perceptible. Finally we must mention the conversations started by adults. In the second part of this work we shall have to investigate the degree to which the starting and development of the individual conversation is to be ascribed to the association of ideas, to perseveration, or to any other theoretical principles.

The child is by no means always equally disposed to talk to the adult present in the same room. When the child has some absorbing occupation he may utter only a single word, or a short sentence, half to himself, half to the other person, and then turn once more to his silent activity. Or the child may ask at intervals a brief question, which should be as briefly answered, so completing the intermezzo. Such utterances can be of value for the interpretation of the child's behaviour, but we will not pursue this line in the present connection. One could note down all the verbal utterances of a child in the course of one day. That might be of distinct service for the purpose of many investigations, but we did not do so because our aim was to limit ourselves to a study of the development of the child's thoughts in conversation. We have therefore included only those conversations which extend at least over a few sentences. In a few exceptional cases we have recorded utterances of the child limited to one sentence, if such appeared to us specially characteristic.

If speech is by far the most important medium of social life, then conversation is the most revealing point at which it appears. Speech is the means of social intercourse which far out-distances all others in efficiency. In conversation we find the most intimate contact of mind with mind, co-operating in a mutual intellectual creative act, and recognizing clearly their social interdependence.[1] To analyse dialogue is therefore to carry on social psychology. Until recently child psychology was scarcely less individualistic than general psychology,[2] but in both fields now there is a strong move towards social psychology.[3] We regard it as probable indeed that the next important progress in social psychology will take in the sphere of child psychology, where many things still are more fluid and consequently more transparent than in the later rigid forms of social life.[4] There is a great deal to be said for Scheler's [5] view that it is not the objective, non-personal experience of the newborn child but rather its expressive experiences that take precedence in its consciousness. The " you consciousness " of the child may at least be born simultaneously with the " I consciousness ", if indeed it is not produced earlier. It is also possible that the " we consciousness "

[1] Litt, Th., *Individuum und Gemeinschaft*, Leipzig und Berlin, 1919.

[2] That applies also to Karl Bühler's otherwise illuminating book : *Die geistige Entwicklung des Kindes*, 4 Aufl., Jena, 1924.

[3] The social psychology of man has recently received great stimulus from animal psychology, which of course goes back to an old tradition of social psychology. We may here recall the investigations of Schjelderup-Ebbe, a student of D. Katz, on the social psychology of birds, upon which the following works are more or less dependent : (a) Katz, D., " Tierpsychologie und Soziologie des Menschen," *Zeitschr. angew. Psychol.*, Bd. 88, 1922. (b) Reiniger, Karl, *Über soziale Verhaltungsweisen in der Vorpubertät*, Wien-Leipzig-New York. (c) Bühler, Charlotte, *Die ersten sozialen Verhaltungsweisen des Kindes*. The valuable work of Bühler, has been published, together with other social studies by Hetzer, Hildegard, and Tudor-Hart, Beatrix, " Soziologische and psychologische Studien über das erste Lebensjahr," *Quellen und Studien zur Jugendkunde*, Herausgegeben von Ch. Bühler, Jena, 1927. Piaget's strongly socialpsychological point of view in the sphere of child psychology is due to folk psychology.

[4] " In the so-called reasoning psychology it is a question of facts which are governed essentially by the social intercourse of men and by their cultural precipitations, chiefly language. They require throughout a social genetic analysis." " Only now do we clearly recognize the social and genetic dependence of the mental world." Krueger, F., " Ueber psychische Ganzheit," *Neue psychologische Studien*, Bd. 1, pp. 7, 11, 1926.

[5] Scheler, M., *Wesen und Formen der Sympathie*, Bonn, 1923.

precedes both the "I" and the "you consciousness".[1] In our opinion the importance of the social-psychological factor in child psychology cannot be overestimated, and it is high time to reorientate the whole of child psychology from the standpoint of social psychology, including also those parts such as perception and volition which seem to form an individualistic reserve.[2] Whatever may be the case before speech is acquired, after its acquisition even the external forms of speech themselves become powerful impulses in the development of the understanding of social relations. It is not for nothing that countless generations have made their social contributions to the instrument of human speech. Even a person who retires from the community into solitude takes with him together with his habit of expressing his thoughts in speech also that of thinking in the "we" or some other social form. The hermit addresses himself to God in religious dialogue. The misanthrope, who avoids his fellows, castigates an imaginary audience or writes for a circle of readers which admittedly he despises, but without whose existence his own position would be meaningless. We all know people who, according to the subject about which they are thinking, imagine other people as actually present and even talk to them, in order to debate and discuss with them. If it is about family affairs, one of the members of the family, usually the husband or wife, is mentally apostrophized. If it concerns the affairs of some society one or more members of the same society will be imagined as supporters, or, more often, as opponents.

---

[1] The "you" is as integral a part of the child's experience as the "I". (Stern, p. 463). Guillaume tries to prove that without the "you consciousness" the "I consciousness" could not develop. Guillaume, Paul, *L'imitation chez l'enfant*, Paris, 1925.—Durkheim and his school in social psychology have stressed the fact that the totality of society is the personal primary in which the individual ego is completely submerged.—In the case of animals living in communities, a completely unreflected "we consciousness" certainly takes precedence over the "I consciousness".

[2] Examples of the impulse given towards setting in motion the will of an adult by the child's will (i.e. the socializing of wills) have been published by us in the *Kindergarten*, Jg. 63, 1922.

C

If it is regarding some scientific treatize then some highly critical colleague is allowed to look over one's shoulder to give his opinion about the work.[1] Janet and Rignano hold that all meditation proceeds from a monologue discussion. Probably it is true to say that whoever is once struck by the miracle of human speech is socialized in his thinking, even though he may have withdrawn from human society.[2] Piaget has made a splendid start in writing the history of the socialization of thought in children. The conversations which follow aim at revealing the importance of the adult in this process. Our important task is to study how the novice in speech makes his earliest attempts to find himself in verbal responses. We mentioned previously the affective-volitional one-word sentences of the young child, which are only uttered in the presence of others, usually to adults familiar to the child. We do not hear them when the child is alone, from which we may deduce that they are socially conditioned. Only in suitable social surroundings does the developing child make this linguistic step forward, whereas experiment has shown that an animal developing in isolation acquires with no delay all those sounds that are used in the animal group to indicate warning, enticement, and so on.[3] When the child enters the first stage of questioning, in which it is curious about the names of things, we note at once that a social factor is converging with the inner maturing process, for there must be someone present who can be questioned. Another person, considered by the child as a superior, must be included in the constellation as stimulus, before any inner questioning attitude can be adopted. Questions are only

[1] In numerous scientific treatises it is obvious at the first glance for whom they were written even though the person concerned is not mentioned in the text.

[2] Natorp is quite right in his statement: " In every heartbeat of our most individual life pulsates, mentally and physically, the life of the totality." Natorp, P., *Sozialpädagogik*, Stuttgart, 1909.

[3] We may mention the exhaustive results obtained by Th. Schjelderup-Ebbe, " Weitere Beiträge zur Sozial- und Individualpsychologie des Haushuhns," *Zeitschr. f. Psychol.*, Bd. 92, 1923.

asked when a reply is confidently expected. That applies to the first questions about the names of objects, to the " Why ? " questions which appear later, and indeed to all types of children's questions which we shall find. Questions and all the conversational attitudes of the child connected with them can only be satisfactorily explained from the standpoint of social psychology.

We mentioned above that the meditations of a solitary thinker, expressed in speech, betray as a rule his social origin. The question now arises as to when and how this habit develops. At present there is little really definite information available towards the solution of this problem. It is very probable that children who have to some extent completed the technique of language acquisition begin to utilize inner speech in those cases where thinking in concrete images for some reason cannot be used. This, of course, cannot be proved at once by directly questioning the child, but it is revealed with some degree of certainty by the child's genuine monologues which the child utters when he really thinks himself alone. In the literature of child psychology we find numerous reports about genuine monologues, some from very early stages of development. E. Köhler often observed monologues by a child of 3 years. Strümpell was able to record monologues of his little daughter when even younger.[1] The assumption seems therefore justified that we have to do with inner speech expressed aloud, and that a great deal is never uttered but is pondered over and decided by this inner speech. The inner speeches will have this in common with those expressed aloud, that the child turns to an imaginary partner and himself carries on the dialogue which develops between the fictitious partner and himself.[2] Who are these partners ? Often

---

[1] Strümpell, L., *Psychologische Pädagogik*, 2 Aufl., Leipzig, 1909.

[2] We append here an example quoted by Groos (*Die Spiele der Menschen*, Jena, 1899), of a dialogue spoken by a little girl of just 5 years old. " Well, sister Olga, so you've come home from your walk ? Do tell me what you saw. A little sheep, a cow, a dog, a horse. Yes, and what else ? Blue bluebells, green cowslips, red leaves ? But there aren't any ; you're telling stories, you know."

they are probably the persons of the child's accustomed environment. Is it permissible to assume that the child visualizes these persons inwardly ? According to some of the observations which we shall communicate later, this does seem to be the case. The conversation-partners in these inner dialogues are most likely the parents, not only because they are with the children more than other people, but also because of the extremely intimate relations in which they stand to the children, a relationship based on authority and love. And so the parents will appear as the most important actors playing opposite the child on the stage of his inner experience. Their role will be usually that of mentors who take up an attitude towards the under-takings the child plans—most frequently as admonishing critics, but occasionally giving encouragement and approval. The voice of conscience is first of all the voice of the parents letting the child know whether his intended action would meet with the approval of the absent parents or not. In an earlier stage of the development of conscience the parent probably comes into the child's mind only after the impulsive action, with its unpleasant consequences, has already taken place. Instead of the parents, or side by side with them, there can appear other people who have regularly had some position of authority in the child's environment. In some cases also people who exist only in the imaginary world of the fairy tale may play their part. If the child receives some religious education, then God may appear as the supreme personal authority who tells the child what is right and wrong. Originally moral conduct is intimately connected with personal authority, for the child cannot comprehend a general principle ; and even if the attempt were made to explain it, the child would immediately convert it into terms of the personal. (Somewhat in the same way as instead of saying, " That isn't done " we say, " Men don't do that.") We shall refer later at greater length to the problems of conscience in connection with our analysis of confessional talk. At this point we only desired briefly to indicate the relationship between the inner life of the child and what is termed as the voice of conscience.

A small circle of people attending a psychological lecture of whose interest we were sure and who we knew possessed the skill necessary for self-observation were asked how they individually behaved during solitary thinking, and whether, in so far as it was thinking carried on by inner speech, they imagined the presence of another person to whom they addressed their words, or whether they spoke to themselves. Our questions were not to be answered at once; we left them a week's time to examine themselves. The result of the self-observation was to be handed in in writing, anonymity being preserved if desired. In order to facilitate mutual understanding the terms "monologue" and "dialogue" thinking were introduced and explained in the preliminary discussion. We endeavoured in this preliminary discussion to avoid all suggestion, and were probably entirely successful, since we ourselves had no very definite expectations about the result of the disclosures. The minority of the persons asked handed in material. Of those we received, three were anonymous. The first of the following replies is from a woman, all the others are from men.

(1) *Hese.*—Usually in monologue, but in dialogue when the task or problem has been brought in from outside. Then in an imaginary conversation with the person who provided the stimulus. As a child she often used to converse with an imaginary figure who became embodied in her favourite doll. If she had suffered an injustice or had an ardent desire for something, then a conversation with God took place, but then God only functioned as an attentive listener. That was when she was 7–9 years old.

(2) *N. N.*—Thinks usually in monologue. A second person to whom he speaks is only imagined when he is repeating something learned by heart. But it is never any definite person.

(3) *Brandt.*—Almost exclusively in monologue. I attribute this to the fact that I had to lecture to students for thirty years. Occasionally I think in dialogue form, e.g. when I am returning from a journey and have bought

something for my wife. Then in my mind I hear her ask a definite question or make some remark or other. In this case memory of previous similar occasions plays a great part.

(4) *N. N.*—Often in dialogue. The partners differ according to the range of thought. Parents, brothers and sisters, children at home, friends, acquaintances, superiors . . . also people who are now dead. I see the partner before me and hear him speak. The conversations can refer to things which happened long ago or to the present time ; they may be mere chats or didactic. Thus, for instance, I go in thought through the fields botanizing with an old colleague and the dialogue then develops.

(5) *Klockmann.*—I very often talk to myself in dialogue form. Then my personal ego is divided into two parts, into a superior or distant part and an inferior or intimate part. The one ego raises a question which is answered by the other. Both correct each other alternately and then come to a mutual end or resolution. In these mutual conclusions the sovereign " We " is usually employed. I am not aware of any dialogue form in which I speak to other people.

(6) *N. N.*—I think mainly in dialogue form. Then I hear inwardly the intonation and usual expressions of the other person. The dialogue form does not always occur with equal clarity, but is very persistent during intensive mental application. The monologue appears in isolated cases, chiefly when thinking of my own person. In the inner dialogue the partner is constantly changing. I cannot say that either sex is predominant. Children are rarely partners, and indeed only when I am preparing lessons. The person imagined as partner is probably determined by the subject-matter being thought of. It is, I think, usually someone with whom one has often before discussed such matters. Especially when in any spoken debate something has made a deep impression on me or if I have been offended or insulted in any way, I find it is usually the people concerned who are the partners during my silent thinking. Intimate friendly relations and mutual or opposed interests can also be the decisive factors in determining a partner. But they are probably in every case people in whom one is interested in some way or other. Even though I know

him personally a person to whom I am quite indifferent will never be my partner in thought.

(7) *Lindemann.*—Often in monologue form, even when he caught himself speaking a few words aloud. A speech to be made at the wedding of a brother-in-law was also prepared in monologue. But thinking in dialogue form does also occur. For instance, when he had heard Mr. G. speak at an election meeting. Then there appeared as partner a schoolmaster who had the same political views as Mr. G. and details were discussed with him. On another occasion Mr. G. himself spoke and he himself made the objections.

(8) *Groth.*—The people to whom I address myself inwardly are clearly imagined. If I have to greet someone I imagine to myself the person and the form of my address. A lecture which I have to deliver is prepared inwardly specifically for an audience imagined as present. If I am to have an interview with a superior, I formulate the sentences in advance, and the superior is imagined in his surroundings. Before I meet in the street people I have seen approaching for some time, the conversation is imagined inwardly just as it takes place later.

We do not intend to enter into a discussion of the above results, as that would lead us too far from our real theme. Our sole object was to illustrate our contention that silent thinking often takes place in dialogue form. On closer investigation we should probably find a rich variety of forms of this inner dialogue. The psychiatrist might with advantage follow them up in his treatment of mental patients.

The study of our dialogues follows two lines : they are to be explained on their formal side and understood from their content. As far as their form is concerned, the dialogues make it necessary for us to explain their structure in terms of as strict a scientific principle as possible. If we admit for the moment the standpoint of classical association psychology, then we shall have to reveal how through the play of the associations familiar to the child on the one hand, and on the other hand of the associations familiar to the adult, there comes into existence finally through the interplay of these two worlds of association every single conversation obtained. Even if we were to broaden the basis of the explanation from which the analysis of the conversations was to proceed by including other explanatory principles, such as the principle of the perseveration of ideas, of deterministic tendencies (Ach), or the theory of specific reaction (Selz), nevertheless the formal side of the problem presented by the conversation could not be abandoned. Let us look into this for a moment. It is highly interesting to set to work applying the well-known explanatory principles to the spontaneous and ample material provided by our conversations ; for the accumulation of a thousand cases of isolated laboratory experiments, such as have been carried out up to now by those dealing with the psychology of memory and thought, can never be directly compared to the analysis of a connected, spontaneous dialogue. We shall discover later the difficulties involved in such an analysis. In numerous cases we have had to explain why the child's conversation at certain places takes just the turn it does, and not some other. That cannot be proved with certainty by means of the principles of explanation used up to the present. But let us suppose we succeeded in completely disentangling the threads which make up the conversations, then only the formal side of the problem would have been solved, not that of the content. This latter problem requires not only the presentation of the content of the child's remarks but also a building up from them of the structure of the world of the child. Before we turn to the question of the fundamental treatment of the content of the conversations it seems fitting to subject the dialogues to investigation from two formal points of view which in our opinion have not yet been esteemed at their proper value in the theories of mental development.

A conversation carried on with a child constitutes a unity from its beginning up to the point where it is concluded by one of the participants to the satisfaction of the other. One is very soon able to judge when the child considers such a conclusion to have been reached. In that case he either ends the conversation by turning away from the adult and devoting himself to some other occupation, or, in a clearly recognizable way, he brings up a new conversational theme. It is of great interest to discover how long a child will stay on a particular theme, that is, the amount of his intellectual staying-power under the demands of conversation. For conversation is not merely in the objective sense a unity which may be investigated by an outsider as a manifestation of the mental processes of those taking part, but it is also experienced by the participants themselves as a unity. The child gets its impression from all the utterances grouped together in the unity. By this we do not imply that in the total experience all the fragments of the dialogue remain equally vivid to the consciousness. For something akin to a law of time-perspective applies in the organization of a speech developing in time, and this law determines that what is farthest away in time is generally less effective. In addition however there is a further distribution of the emphasis within the whole, according to the importance of the individual parts of the conversation for the idea being developed in it. In certain cases therefore parts of the conversation more distant in time could get special stress. As far as we know no investigation along this line has yet been made in general psychology. The performances considered here differ from the experiments on the so-called memory span by the fact that they are not restricted in time to a period limited essentially to the present ; and they differ from the tests in which an account of the main parts of a story is required by the fact that both the productive as well as the reproductive factors are brought into operation. Our conversations allow us to get closer from an almost totally neglected side to the peculiar relations which exist between mechanical memory and reproductive-productive intelligence.

Whenever mathematical functions have been used in psychology to represent the regularities noted (and this has been the case particularly in connection with sensation and perception and in memory research) it is always continuous functions that have been used. By this recognition is given to the continuity of mental functions, or at least to the functional relationships between mental phenomena, at least for those branches in which mathematical formulae have been utilized. But even where such formulations have not been actually used, at least the dominance of the principle of continuity in the mental sphere and in its closely connected physiological spheres has been tacitly admitted. The determining factor was probably the method of observation in the inorganic and organic natural sciences, on which experimental psychology was in the first place based. We do not dispute that the stream of consciousness flows to a great extent continuously, and that its law can be deduced, if not with the approximation to accuracy so fondly cherished by an earlier optimism, at least in principle through definite analytical functions. But on the other hand there are in the coming and going of mental images gaps whose laws, to continue in mathematical terminology, are only to be approached by means of arithmetical functions.[1] The deeper we have delved into the mental development of the child, the clearer do we see that the principle of continuity

[1] The first to draw attention to these relationships was probably W. G. Alexejeff in his treatise, " Die arithmologischen und wahrschein-lichkeitstheoretischen Kausalitäten als Grundlagen der Strümpellschen Klassifikationen der Kinderfehler," *Zeitschr. Philos. u. Pädag.*, vol. 3, 1906. A. Bethe and E. Woitas, " Funktionswechsel nervöser Zentren nach Amputation von Gliedmassen," *Bericht über die ges. Physiologie u. exp. Pharmakologie*, Bd. 32, 1925, have shown that the organs of water-beetles, dor-beetles (*geotropes stercorarius*), and spiders (shepherd spiders, *phalangium opilio*) take on quite new functions, never exercised before, and making possible a logical total behaviour of the creature, if the animals are deprived of various members through amputation. Here before our very eyes we watch the behaviour of new creation, which works completely uncontinuously, under the pressure of an entirely new situation, due to the mutilation of the organism as a whole. The assumption that the co-ordination of movement takes place according to a plan deeply rooted in the anatomical distribution of the nerve centres cannot be upheld, maintain A. Bethe and E. Woitas. " The old saw that nature makes no leaps forward did not become false for the first time when the quantum theory was propounded. If nature took no leaps forward, there could not possibly be the great agreement prevailing in general in the systems of animal, vegetable and mineral kingdoms." Petzold, T. Komplex und Begriff, *Zeitschr. f. Psychol.*, Bd. 102, p. 282, 1927

is not sufficient to reveal it and that the decisive progress takes place as distinct leaps forward. The continuity method of consideration does perhaps apply for changes in the child's performances which are quantitative in nature, but is certainly to be rejected for the development of characteristics which are qualitatively different. Therefore we consider that the designation of development as " gradual " so popular in works on child psychology should be altered to " sudden ". Somewhere in the individual life of the child consciousness flashes for the first time into being, and, unless one is desirous of taking refuge in unfounded metaphysical speculations, there can be no question of a continuous transition process from the unconscious. Every transition from waking to sleeping and vice versa takes place suddenly ; every new sense-perception of the child appears abruptly in the child's mental life and is not to be explained from purely psychical causality. The feelings of jealousy, sympathy, pride, and all others that can be distinguished must be produced for the first time suddenly from the corresponding situation. Let us take an example from the sphere of the taking up of intellectual attitudes by the child. Whoever is of the opinion that a judgment is qualitatively different from an association of ideas (on this point, with K. Bühler we agree with Brentano's view) must, when faced by the fact that the new-born child cannot, whereas the 2-year-old can, adopt a critical attitude to things, admit that the child accomplished the new performance at some time or other without there being any continuous transition.[1]

[1] Dallenbach has reported the sudden realization of the meaning of the word " opposite " in a conversation with his six-year-old son. " John, do you know what ' opposite ' means ? " " No." " Yes, you do : tell me what the opposite of good is." " Boy." " No, that is not the opposite of good. Now tell me, what the opposite of big is." " Man." " Wrong again. The opposite of good is bad, of big, little. Do you understand ? " " Yes." " Good, then tell me what the opposite of black is." " White." " Of long ? " " Short." " Of thick ? " " Thin." " Of big ? " " Little." " Of bad ? " " Good." So it proceeded, without mistake. Dallenbach, "A note on the immediacy of understanding a relation," *Psychol. Forsch.*, vol. 7, 1926.

K. Bühler is one of those psychologists who have drawn considerable attention to the principle of discontinuity in connection with problems of child psychology. But he fails to make the principle really fruitful by neglecting to apply it to special cases of child development. Bühler bases his considerations about the process of release in the organism on the work of v. Kries, and on the well-known lecture of Strumpf on the idea of evolution in contemporary philosophy.[1] Strumpf maintains in this lecture that the individual qualities of sensation must have leaped into existence suddenly, as we simply cannot conceive the transition from one sense quality to another. He comes to the conclusion that a continuously progressive development on the physical side is accompanied by a discontinuous development on the mental side ; that corresponding to gradual and quantitative difference on the one side we can have qualitative and specific difference on the other. Bühler restricts the consideration of discontinuity to the problems of the origin of sensation, without, as was only to be expected, coming to any satisfactory conclusion. " No one has up to now been able to answer the question, from what biological necessity sensations proceed." [2]   In a criticism of Bühler's book we emphasized the necessity of asserting the claims of the principle of discontinuing in a more general form in child psychology.[3] H. Werner has recently confessed himself a fervent believer in this principle of development. " It has been (erroneously) thought that mental development is inseparably connected with mathematical continuity, and that development could be at once symbolized by the form of a mathematical line. . . . And

---

[1] Published in Stumpf, C., *Philosophische Reden und Vorträge*, Leipzig, 1910.

[2] In the study of the sensations of vibration (Katz, D., *Der Aufbau der Tastwelt*, Leipzig, 1925), we have an attempt to reveal (previously unheeded) relationships between sensations. The sensations of vibration have in their form and function an astoundingly close relation to the sensations of hearing, while they are quite different from them in quality.

[3] *Zeitschr. Psychol.*, vol. 86, 1921.

yet the theory of continuity is maintained by hardly a single biologist. One is perhaps ready to admit the fact of a new creative performance in the field of sensations and their development, but as soon as one considers higher functions such as ideation and thinking, the problem becomes confused . . . (in reality development takes place) in the form of typical mental stages, the higher of which is to be regarded as a new creative performance as compared to the lower." [1]

The fact that in general the principle of continuity has taken precedence in scientific thinking for the understanding and explanation of natural processes must of course find its explanation deep down in the natural tendencies of human thinking. In biology the microscopic observation of the processes of development brought about the application of the principle of continuity. It was the new atomic theory (Quantum theory) which for the first time made it possible for the physicist to admit the existence of discontinuous processes also in inorganic nature. If we consider that neither the chemist's retort nor the physicist's precision-apparatus for the recognition of physical chemistry processes gives such fine reactions as the processes of consciousness (this consideration is independent of any special idea one may have of the relation of body-mind) then it will not seem too fantastic to perceive a certain relationship between the psychological principle of discontinuity and the basic principle of the quantum theory. Hempelmann has recently done this in considering the origin of consciousness. " Certain absolute quanta of some material kind or other must always come together if a process is to take place. The seemingly continuous processes proceed in reality by stages (Quantum theory). That is shown by the presence of the stimulus threshold in physiology and psychology. If the physiological processes in the cortex overstep the threshold by even the smallest possible quantity, intensity or complexity of structure then consciousness is present." [2]

---

[1] Werner, H., *Einführung in die Entwicklungspsychologie*, p. 14 f., 1926 (Henceforth quoted as Werner).

[2] Hempelmann, F., *Tierpsychologie*, p. 621, Leipzig, 1926.

In our opinion the doctrine of apsychonomous events can be classed as a general and the doctrine of perseverations within the psychology of memory as a special concession to the principle of discontinuity.[1] As the analyses of our conversations will show, both theories reveal themselves to be applicable in a high degree to child psychology. Indeed one is almost surprised that they were not formulated here instead of in general psychology.[2] This doctrine of perseveration was opposed by investigators such as Ebbinghaus, Kiesow, and Wundt under the dogma, " No reproduction without association." Their opposition is based fundamentally on a disinclination to assume discontinuity in mental events. They preferred to take refuge in the assumption of most improbable associative connecting links which remained undetected. Wundt's resistance to the possibility of perseverative reproduction arose from the fear of assuming along with it a causeless happening, which would be a contradiction of the principle of causality as applied to the mental sphere. But logically discontinuous happening by no means implies causeless happening.

In his investigations into the progress of speech in children Stern came very near to assuming a discontinuous development. Helen Keller in her autobiography gives a very impressive description of the moment when the value of the symbols in the group of letters she was touching dawned upon her. Here we have a really classical case of a gap in the series of mental events. But it was not her outstanding intelligence which played the chief part in the form of speech development which took place, for entirely similar results have been observed in the case of other deaf, dumb, and blind children learning to speak, as for instance those in

[1] For the conception of apsychonomous events cf. Müller, G. E., *Zur Analyse der Gedächtnistätigkeit und des Vorstellungsverlaufes*, part 3, Leipzig, 1913. The doctrine of the perseveration of ideas in its first form was developed by Müller and Pilzecker, 1900.

[2] Ach has applied the doctrine of perseveration to child psychology. Ach, N., Kühle, E., and Passarge, E., *Beiträge zur Lehre von der Perseveration*, Leipzig, 1926.

the Nowawes institution near Berlin.[1]   A whole series of pertinent examples. " At such moments when one becomes strangely conscious of the discrepancy between present perception and the previous conception of a state of affairs, other inner processes must also be taking place. In a similar drastic way present and past must fall apart " (p. 59). " It is impossible not to think that the distance between Ann's physical and mental capacity has suddenly, at a bound, become still greater " (p. 64). " It is certain that at such moments clearly the correct convergence for the birth of wit is afforded " (p. 144).

If we seek in general psychology for examples of processes in which the investigator was struck by their discontinuity we shall have to refer to the category of " Aha "-experiences laid down by Bühler in his experiments on the psychology of thought.[2]   Corresponding to these we have in animal psychology the sudden solutions of problems by W. Köhler's anthropoid apes.[3]   The psychology of religion could not fail to notice the great significance of sudden religious conversions, the special character of which gave rise to the use of terms like " regeneration " and " rebirth " (W. James, E. O. Starbuck).

When we come to analyse our conversations we shall endeavour to make this principle of the discontinuity of development yield fruit. This will be—in contrast to those mental processes which proceed almost entirely reproductively—chiefly where a new problem is solved, that is where the child behaves as a creator of new things. In the child chance acts as the stimulus to production behaviour much more frequently than in the adult.[4]

---

[1] Cf. Katz, D., *Psychologie und mathematischer Unterricht*, p. 89, Leipzig, 1913.

[2] Bühler, K., " Tatsachen und Probleme zu einer Psychologie der Denkvorgänge," *Arch. f. d. ges. Psychol.*, vol. 9, 1907.

[3] Köhler, W., *Intelligenzprüfungen an Anthropoiden*, 2 ed., Berlin, 1922.

[4] He draws attention to the important investigations into the importance of chance for productive thought carried out by Selz, O., *Zur Psychologie des produktiven Denkens und des Irrtums*, Bonn, 1922.

If an object lesson on this problem is required, observe a child for a short time when he is playing with building blocks. Purely accidental positions which the blocks have assumed cause the child to see entirely new possibilities of arrangement and utilization, and spur on his imagination to still higher achievements. But, however accidental the origin of the outer constellation of stimuli, one must not imagine the child as an equally accidental and passively reacting quantity. His reaction to the new performance bears the stamp of the greatest activity. This is particularly clear when the child pushes forward into original unexpected results. But of course it does not occur only in that instance ; rather is it true that the miracle of creative achievement is performed every day and every hour of the child's development. In the process of adaptation, whether it lies in the sphere of sense perception, of motor reaction, of imagination, or of intellect, every new situation demands a new creative activity even though reproductive elements also play their part in some degree towards the total performance. Where could we find in life such a repetition of a situation where adaptation is attained with exactly the same means as before ? Every real step forward the child makes in the acquisition of knowledge, however small it may be, takes place discontinuously. We are in agreement with Koffka's statement that " Discontinuity is present at that point in the learning process where the (desired) performance is accomplished for the first time." Koffka is quite right in distinguishing the problem of achievement from that of memory, for the former takes place suddenly, whilst the latter is gradually perfected.[1] When the child achieves something spontaneously we can speak of discontinuous progress to an even greater degree than when we induce it to perform an action desired by us. We have principally to look for discontinuity at those points in the recorded conversations where the child asks questions which are

---

[1] Koffka, K., *Psychologie. Lehrbuch der Philosophie. Die Philosophie in ihren Einzelgebieten*, herausgegeben von M. Dessoir, p. 567, Berlin.

called forth by the consciousness of a lack or a gap which needs filling, or by the consciousness of an inhibition or obstruction which demands removal.

Inanimate nature knows no creative force. The scientist may indeed discover there new chemical elements and new physical-chemical energies, but no new elements come into being and no new types of energy are developed. Conditions in the animate living world are quite different. Life does not repose within itself, it is never concluded and develops from itself new forms and forces. It is possible that there are dynamic periods when its formative capacity is greater than at other times, but in general we may say that the power of mental productivity only comes to an end at death. We have stated that no physical-chemical method affords so intimate a glimpse into what is happening to living substances as the processes of consciousness. And if that is true then we may justly hope that consciousness will provide the most accurate information about the methods of adaptation in the living organism and about its creative forces.[1] In Bühler's " step by step " (Stufen) theory we find an important contribution to a theory of the creative powers of consciousness. According to this theory the birth of new types of functions takes place when it is a question of complying suddenly and completely with new and unfamiliar demands (Bühler, p. 25). This theory will certainly hold good for many cases, but it is conceivable that, considering the high level which the human mind has now reached, the development from within will be carried on even without such a biological compulsion. We have only to think of the discovery of abstruse scientific methods

---

[1] It is only following the line of these ideas that in order to confirm Lamarck's hypothesis of the heredity of acquired qualities, the clumsy methods of external operative interference are now being dropped and instead the attempt is being made to train successive generations of a species of animal under investigation to a definite mode of behaviour towards sense-impressions, cf. W. McDougall, " An Experiment for the Testing of the Hypothesis of Lamarck," *Brit. Journ. of Psychol.*, vol. 17, 1927.

and of the setting up of new standards of value in all spheres of artistic activity.

In Köhler's experiments a new achievement is wrung from the apes under our very eyes : under the compulsion of the situation the animal performs something which it had never before been able to do. We become witnesses of a discontinuous leap forward of animal intelligence. It is not a question of the absolute level of the new performance ; the important point is that in the system concerned the new performance goes beyond the former level. Koffka has made determined efforts to transfer this theory into child psychology by affirming that in the behaviour of the individual something fundamentally new can occur, something which is not entirely dependent on heredity and environment.[1] In general developmental psychology Werner has propounded a similar theory " Development means the formation of something new and creative change " (Werner, p. 17).

The non-closure of creative development renders difficult any prophecy either qualitative or quantitative about the probable course of events in the mental sphere. The physicist is able to predict the course of a laboratory experiment with perfect accuracy. And the meteorologist is content with his far smaller number of accurate predictions only because he is not able to take note of all the conditions which influence the weather, and not because there are any other than these fundamental mechanical ones so well known to him to be taken into account. The experimental conditions in the laboratory can so govern the course of mental events that the psychologist leaves the meteorologist far behind in accuracy of prediction. But where we come face to face with the possibility of new mental creations, all prophecy is useless. Who would dare to maintain that no new modes of sensation are to be gained from the mind or that there is no possibility of any genuine new achievement in the realm of feeling and intellect ? In individual mental life we need only an odour not previously smelled for a new

[1] Koffka, K., *Die Grundlagen der psychischen Entwicklung*, 2nd ed., Osterwieck, 1925.

quality, even if not a new mode of sensation to cross the threshold of our consciousness. Does not a new work of art reveal to us new emotional experiences ? " By new compositions feelings of a depth and variety never previously experienced by anyone are aroused."[1] When in a mathematics lecture the "limes-concept" dawns on a person for the first time, a new intellectual creative process is performed. In the light of the views we have just put forward, the psychological conception of causality stands in need of revision.[2] In physics too, with its recent developments concerning atomic-structure, there has sprung up an extremely lively discussion, by no means concluded, about the concept of causality.[3]

Let us assume that the ideal has been attained in the explanation of our conversations along the lines which we have indicated and that we have succeeded in unravelling the tangled threads of association, perseveration, and the other processes which must and did lead to their production. Does the psychologist's work end there ? No, for such a task could also have been performed without our being obliged to discuss the content of the conversations any differently from a more or less accidental material : this purely formal investigation could have been carried out with much the same result on other conversations of our children, not recorded here, or on any conversation of any children, even children of a different race. Such an investigation would give us information about the course of those configurative formative-processes in children, but nothing further. We should learn nothing about the special life-form (Lebensform) and life-content (Lebensinhalt) which are revealed to us from the recorded conversations of the two children who differ so considerably in character. The contrast between the two methods can also be shown by an

---

[1] Kries, J. v., *Wer ist musikalisch ?* Berlin, 1926.

[2] According to the previously mentioned work of Alexejeff necessity and fatal unavoidability are characters of analytical causalities : individuality and freedom accompany arithmological causalities.

[3] Cf. Planck, M., " Physikalische Gesetzlichkeit im Lichte neuerer Forschung," *Naturwissenschaften*, 1926, No. 13. Jordan, " Kausalität und Statistik in der modernen Physik," *Naturwissenschaften*, 1927, No. 5.

example from general psychology. In textbooks on that subject there is scarcely anything to be found dealing with the cultural content of the human beings whose psychology is being revealed. The textbook of psychology written by a German and referring to Germans is in its essentials exactly the same as the textbook of his Japanese colleague, writing in Japanese. There is no mention of the concrete values recognized by the people whose mental life is being investigated, but only of the attitude adopted to abstract values ; the content of thought is not taken into account, but merely thought in general. In fact everything which makes up the essential content of the culture of a human being of this or that country, his life-content (Lebensinhalt) slips through the meshes of the general psychologist's investigating-net, and so social and cultural psychology, ethnology, and sociology are left to deal with the things neglected by general psychology. It is from those branches of science that we glean our information about what belongs essentially to the psychology of a human being : that is, about the things which really make up the content of his experience, what values govern him, what thoughts he has, and in general the outline of his conception of the world.[1] In child psychology the distribution of labour has not yet progressed so far, and so the child-psychologist is compelled to act as cultural and social psychologist, ethnologist, etc., during his investigations. Everything concerned with the content side of the child mind could be grouped together under the heading " child culture ". In our conversations this culture of the children is disclosed to us in both form and content. The task of revealing it would not be affected even if the explanatory efforts should for some reason completely fail in their object.

Every child begins in his own way—one that is clearly recognizable after he had acquired his mother tongue—

---

[1] E. Spranger, *Psychologie des Jugendalters*, 3 Aufl., Leipzig, 1925, has made the most noteworthy attempt to describe the psychology of youth from this new point of view.

to build up for himself his view of the world
(Weltanschauung). However primitive and labile in
structure it may be, it is there. It is determined by what
the child makes of the material present in his environment.
And therefore the subject-matter of the conversations
constantly taking place in the child's environment is bound
to be of the utmost importance. Let us take this statement first of all in its truest general sense. A child growing
up in Rostock will of course hear chiefly about the streets
and places and surroundings of Rostock rather than, say,
of Berlin. On the coast the sea and ships will be spoken
about oftener than they are inland.[1] Thus the content
of the child world of ideas receives a regional, geographical
coloration. Numerous experiments have been carried out
to analyse the ideation equipment of children reaching school
age, and even though the attitude towards the experiments
has been almost always atomistic, yet there is no doubt
about the justification and necessity of the investigation
into the content of the children's thought in its dependence
on environment. The content of its thought is determined
not only by geographical considerations but to a far greater
extent by the family circle. In a middle-class family the
mental nourishment the child derives from the conversation
is quite different from that obtained in a working-class
family, leaving out of account for the time being any discussion as to their respective values. In a religious family
the child becomes familiar with religious ideas earlier
than in a family which excludes religion from its conversational topics. So each family produces a different mental
idiom and a different child's world of thought.[2] The

---

[1] That is clearly shown by children's dreams. Cf. Carla Raspe,
" Untersuchungen über Kinderträume," *Zeitschr. päd. Psychol.*, vol. 25,
1924.

[2] The first school-year in the elementary school reveals a relative lack
of uniformity in individualities ; the most varied kinds of environment
have acted upon the newcomers to school-life, and school at first performs
a levelling function. A. Busemann, *Ueber die Seelengestalt des Volks-
schülers*, Erziehung, vol. 192.

child adopts the values and points of view of his environment and changes them in his own way, modifying them
according to his powers. The fact that there is not always
a deeper insight to be perceived in these modifications
is less striking than the courage with which the child sets
about the task.[1] There is no adult whose world is quite
free from pictures of his desires, and children of the age
with which we are dealing live in a world completely
dominated by pictures of wishes and future hopes. But we
shall also have to record the existence of genuine problems
in the " Weltanschauung " of our elder child, the metaphysical problems of cosmogeny and theology thrust themselves
into his world of thought. Just as in the case of the adult
so also in children there is no clear-cut division between
the life-content and life-form, but they are to a large extent
mutually conditioned. The child's scale of values, which
may be very arbitrary, determines the wish-pictures. There
is a very close connection between the wishes of the child
and his way of magical thinking. The magical apprehension
of his environment is a fundamental part of the child's
life-form, and there is no doubt from our experience that
every child who slips into the magical way of thinking
would remain for ever hopelessly bound to it but for the
intervention of the environment. For we see this actually
occur in the case of the child of the primitive man, who
himself thinks magically.[2]

Conversations with adults introduce the child into the
world of " objective mind ". However slight at first may
be the pressure towards the recognition of the objectively

[1] " The child cannot learn to drive a car like grown-ups but that does
not prevent him in the least from solving the problem in his own way."
Martha Muchow, " Beiträge zur psychologischen Charakteristik des
Kindergarten- und Grundschulalters," *Pädagogisch-psychologische Schriften
des allgemeinen deutschen Lehrerinnenvereins*, No. 3, p. 12, Berlin, 1926.

[2] Carla Raspe has investigated magical thinking in older children in
her work on the child's self-observation and theory-forming. *Zeitschr.
angew. Psychol.*, vol. 23, p. 320 ff., 1924. Werner has gone into magical
thinking more thoroughly and in greater detail in his above-mentioned
work.

valid conditions to which he is subjected, the child has begun to think conceptionally and continues more and more to do so. In numerous examples from the conversations we shall discover how notably different in form the child's way of thinking is from that of adults and we shall have to characterize these forms. Nevertheless in our deductions we shall not be able entirely to dispense with the standard of logical correspondence to fact, for logical thinking is really not only the aim of education but the pressure in (natural) development also tends towards this goal. With the unfolding of autonomous thinking the purely biological method of approach to the child's mental development must be abandoned. This method has proved extremely fruitful in setting up parallels from animal psychology. The applicability of structure-psychological points of view to the mental life of the child appears to us as vindicated in so far as it seeks to grasp super-individual " sense-processes " (Sinnzusammenhänge) and is orientated round them. We have an obvious example of this in the comprehension of the simplest arithmetical relationship. But it is not so easy to apply these structural-psychological points of view in order to establish the connection between subjective functional states. The data obtained by child-psychology on this subject up to the present cannot be considered as final. The difference between an understanding and an explanatory attitude towards the material of child psychology is not thereby removed, as indeed we ourselves have recognized *de facto* in earlier publications. But we shall not yield to the temptation to undertake a critical examination of this problem which is causing such a stir in all psychological circles. It is of course necessary to have undertaken a discussion of such a " fundamental " question but it is much more necessary to have attempted to construct something on the new foundations. In the discussion of the individual conversations there will be much to say to an understanding psychologist and we believe that it is from this very point of view of understanding on the part of the child (we must also include understanding on the part of the animal [1]) that we may obtain new stimuli for a discussion of the question of understanding.

We may add a few details about the method of recording the conversations. Often they were noted down in an abbreviated form by one of us, whilst the other was chatting to the children. Occasionally they were taken down by the nursery-maid whilst both of us were engaged in the conversation ; in these cases she would sit in the next room, with the door open. If the nurse had been seen writing in the same room it would have appeared unusual to the children, whereas they were quite accustomed to seeing one of us engaged in writing while the other was chatting to them. We can state with absolute certainty that the children never imagined any connection between their speaking and our taking notes, and with equal certainty that they have up to the present day not the slightest idea that they are the chief characters in a published work. So it is really obvious that the children can never be accused of trying to shine or be " literary " in their conversations. For many of the short conversations no notes were required. They could easily be remembered and were written down immediately the conversation was ended. But my wife soon developed a surprising skill in reproducing even the longer conversations in most accurate detail from memory, and these too were then at once recorded. So the conversations are word-for-word reproductions of the originals. Here and there in the reconstruction of the conversation from the notes or in its reproduction from memory some slight change in the order of words may have crept in, or some other expression may have replaced the one used by the child, but the sense of the child's utterance has in no case been affected thereby. The expert will at once be able to see from the structure of the sentences how closely these utterances of our children correspond to their age. Although

[1] Cf. Katz, D., " Charakterologie und Tierpsychologie," *Jahrb. der Charakterologie*, Berlin, 1927.

we have endeavoured to be as accurate as possible it must be remembered that literal accuracy was not so absolutely essential here as it is when a child's first sounds or sentences are being recorded. The various ways in which an adult is able to give expression to his thoughts is due to the emancipation of the process of thinking from purely linguistic hindrances, an emancipation which has already begun at the age of three when the child has to a large extent ended its purely external acquisition of speech. In view of this, our attempts to present an absolutely word-for-word rendering of the conversations were perhaps somewhat exaggerated.

As neither the phonetics nor the grammar of child-language was our concern, we have not attempted to give in the text a phonetically correct reproduction of the particular dialect of the children, neither have we paid attention to the more trivial grammatical errors they made. The trouble involved in attaining these ends during the first recording of the conversations would have been out of all proportion to the value of the results obtained. Concerning our children's dialect we need merely state that the language of Fritz Reuter, the Mecklenburg poet, has had a great influence. This is a confirmation of many previous experiences where the local dialect, by means of servants, playmates, and acquaintances has more influence on the speech of young children than the dialect spoken in the closer family-circle. We have only departed from our principle of not recording grammatical errors in the text, inserting instead the correct forms, when, as in a few instances provided by our younger child, we considered the original form especially instructive. The elder boy scarcely ever made such mistakes. Indeed, he possessed an extremely good vocabulary—better than his brother at the same age, and revealed greater certainty and skill in verbal expression. Anyone whose main interest is phonetics and the obtaining of absolutely accurate literal recordings of dialogue must have resource to technical apparatus, such as for instance the parlograph ;

but, in view of the results of experiments with a parlograph in the psychological institute here, we can state that in those circumstances one can never be sure of obtaining a natural verbal utterance either of child or adult. The use of a gramophone would lead to a dearly bought apparent accuracy. The problem we are concerned with here does not demand phonetic accuracy, though of course anyone desirous of undertaking phonetic studies of child language will find accurate recording instruments indispensable.

Anyone who reads the following conversations in the same way as he reads conversation in literature, that is without laying stress on the scientific side, will doubtless be able to get a vivid and realistic picture of the two children taking part. No psychographic work, however exhaustive and artistic, could portray the children as plastically and faithfully as they appear in the direct speech of their own verbal utterances, in which are mirrored both their personality and their conception of the world. And does not this use of direct speech constitute one of the main charms of the Platonic dialogues ? The influence they have had is most intimately connected with the suggestive form of the dialogue, in which the exponents of various ideas, above all Socrates, are taking part. The fact that Socrates, so to speak, addresses himself to us and acts upon us with all the arts of oratory makes him by far the most living of all philosophers. The Platonic dialogues are artificial conversations, but we say to ourselves that clever men might very well have conversed together in just this way about matters of philosophy in which they were vitally interested. The unprejudiced statement of the various points of view represented, the skilful interplay of argument and counter-argument, the way in which the conversation is steered to a definite goal, all this produces an effect comparable to the pleasure of listening to a magnificent symphony. This vivid method of developing ideas, scarcely possible in any other form, has caused the Platonic dialogues to be used often as a pattern for the portrayal of processes of thought in artistic dialogue both in philosophy and elsewhere.[1] In view of the wealth of psychological material to be found in conversations it is to be deplored that literal conversations for the thousand and one opportunities afforded by the daily life of civilized and natural man have been so sparingly used as sources for investigation. Here we make a beginning with conversations from the nursery, and we are at present engaged in collecting the further conversations of our growing children. Teachers in all kinds of schools have numerous opportunities of getting literal records of conversations with their own pupils. Conversations in lessons having a fixed aim as well as informal chats with no scientific purpose are equally welcome.[2] But in order to draw up a complete scheme of classification of conversations, it would be desirable to obtain records of conversations between adults and discussions in learned circles and societies. If we are not mistaken an almost inexhaustible supply of material is here waiting to be revealed by social psychology.

[1] We may mention Berkeley and Leibniz as examples of philosophers who have written treatises in dialogue form.

[2] F. E. Otto Schultze, *Grundlegung der Pädagogik*, Langensalza, 1926, records literally conversations between teachers and pupils. The work of R. von Krafft-Ebing, *Hypnotische Experimente*, 4 Aufl., Leipzig, 1926, gives in detail a dialogue between doctor and patient. Literal records of conversations between medical authorities and their patients could have a high practical and educational value.

PART I

The individual conversations are given in the exact
sequence in which they were recorded, numbered 1–141
for the purpose of speedy reference in the general discussion
which takes place in Part II of this work. In addition to
the date of each conversation we have given in each case
a fairly close indication of the time of day, which, as we
shall see, is not without its influence on the inclination
of the children to reply in some definite way, or even at all.
At the head of many of the conversations are to be found
also such brief descriptions of the situation as we considered
important for the understanding of the conversation.
We have, more rarely, introduced into the text in parentheses
brief explanatory remarks concerning what the child said
and, more frequently, remarks referring to changes in the
initial situation or to actions of the persons taking part
in the conversation. We found it more practical to include
these remarks in the text rather than in the discussion
immediately following. Finally there are in the text, also
in parentheses, small letters of the alphabet, by means of
which reference is made in the discussion to that portion
of the dialogue immediately preceding them. We have not
used these letters when the conversations are quite short
or where there could be no possible confusion about the part
of the dialogue under discussion. As a rule the point at
which the speaker—child or adult—goes over to a quite
new thought is indicated in the text by a dash. Naturally
the discussion could not deal with all possible theoretical
points of view ; any attempt to do that would have filled
several volumes of this size. For there is no important

question of child psychology which could not be touched upon somehow in discussing these conversations. As we analysed our dialogues we realized with regret that so many questions of general psychology which it would be of interest and profit to apply to problems of child psychology still remain unsolved.

The most important participants in the conversations were :—

1. The children's father, henceforth referred to as F. Addressed by the children as Papa.

2. The children's mother, henceforth referred to as M. Addressed by the children as Mama.

3. The children's grandmother, the mother of M., referred to as G.

4. Wilhelm Theodor, called Theodor, referred to as T. T. was born on 8th November, 1920 ; his age can be calculated in all cases from the date above each conversation.

5. Julius Gregor, called Julius, referred to as J. He was born on 6th July, 1922. The abbreviations of the children's names will not be used when they are addressed.

6. The nurse, Olga, addressed by the children as Auntie Olga, referred to as O. She has been with us since November, 1925.

7. The maid, Elli, called by the children simply Elli. Referred to as E. With us since September, 1925.

In the conversations other persons are mentioned, both children and adults, relatives, or acquaintances of the children. These are referred to in the conversations by the names by which the children called them : their family name is abbreviated.

I

9.10.25. Morning in bed. The children are both looking at the coloured illustrations in a cookery-book.

T. : " Mama, here is the cellar, here are roots and fruit for the winter." (To J.) : " I suppose you want to eat meat again ? " (a).

J. : " Yes."

T. : " Which do you like best in the book, the meat or the dwarfs ? "

J. : " Meat *and* dwarfs." (*b*).

T. : " I like everything in this book best." (*c*).

J. (turning over the pages. A coloured illustration of meat and cakes appears, and causes J. to act as if he had something in his mouth which he was chewing) : " Mama, just look."

J. : " Cakes."

T. : " Pestol." (*d*).

J. : " Pestol."

T. : " Pestol."

J. : " Pestol."

T. : " The dwarf is laughing."

J. : " I think he's pleased over us." (*e*).

T. : " The book is slipping off, it will have to be stuck." (The corners of the cookery-book were coming off through the children frequently using it).

J. : " It must be stuck. Mama, a dwarf."

T. : " Then a beetle. The book is slipping."

J. : " A naughty book, a nice book." (*f*).

T. : " He (i.e. the dwarf) is pouring soup."

J. : " He is pouring soup."

M. (reading aloud from the book) : " The meat must be covered with water."

J. (peers into the book) : Where is it covered ? I can't see it." (*g*).

Discussion.—The cookery-book, with its numerous coloured illustrations, amongst which were many dwarfs, as helpers of the housewife, had become at this time as it were the children's favourite picture-book which they turned to again and again. It was considered a special privilege to be allowed to look at it in the mornings in bed. Thus the situation is general. Now to a consideration of the individual parts of the conversation. (*a*) To make this question clear, we must relate some additional facts. J. is very fond of meat. We have seen him pick up from his plate a large piece of meat and bite into it before we had time to cut it into small pieces, or he has suddenly seized a whole sausage from the table and buried his teeth in it. He likes potatoes, but no vegetables except carrots. This taste which he has retained up to the present is doubtless inborn, just in the same way, and to the same extent, as T. is of decidedly vegetarian tastes. In their earliest years we saw to it that both boys were fed as much as possible on a vegetarian diet. When a little meat was added as an extra, T. did not exactly refuse it, but he was quite indifferent. The elder boy likes the most varied kinds of puddings, vegetables, especially raw tomatoes, all kinds of fruit in season, and almost every sort of mild cheese. But his brother J. has quite different tastes. At first he shared his brother's delight in puddings, but very soon after he had tasted meat he came to prefer it, to such an extent that we had to make an effort to oppose this tendency. As we have said, he would eat no vegetables except carrots, which he liked probably because they were the first he tasted (when about eight months old). It would have been quite impossible to make him eat raw tomatoes. He would not touch many kinds of fruit, of which T. was passionately fond, e.g. grapes. He also had no liking for cheese. It seems as if T's tastes, which probably differ from those of the average of children of his age more than do J's, had been strongly influenced by his mother, who once when a student lived on a vegetarian diet for two to three years. J's appetite for meat is also perhaps rather greater than is usual for a child of his age ; it may be that he is rather following in his father's footsteps. Questions of appetite and taste, the latter of course in the biological and not in the atomistic sense, deserve more attention from child psychologists than they have yet received, for as far as our knowledge of the literature goes they have been almost entirely neglected in investigations into child psychology, just as they have in those of adults. Quite apart from all theoretical considerations about appetite, of which we have singled out one concerned with the problem of heredity, these things are of immediate practical importance. The morning rolls are spread for T. with cheese, for J. with sausage, and on picnics when the food is all in one package the greatest care has to be taken to

see that no confusion occurs in the distribution of the food.
Because of such happenings, T. is aware of J's particular
tastes and in question (*a*) is trying to tease him. (*b*) This
answer is just as characteristic of childish logic as the
question to which it is the answer. Meat and dwarfs :
what adult would dare to draw comparisons of value between
two such uncommensurable things. And what adult would
think of the solution which J. finds. Meat *and* dwarfs are
liked best, i.e. both are liked extremely well, he would not
like to be without either the one or the other.[1] The child's
logic finds no obstacle in the fact that several superlatives
side by side are impossible. Something similar is probably
the cause of the thoughtlessness of the adult who, overcome
each time by his last feelings and impressions, declares
that he has never enjoyed himself so much in his life as
at the dance he has just left. T's decision (*c*), that he likes
everything in the cookery-book best of all arises through
making " best of all " equal in meaning to " extremely
well ". (*d*) Here we have the formation of a new word,
whose roots we are not able to indicate.[2] The word, meaningless to us, is repeated by J., who also reveals in other
conversations a frequently necessary tendency to imitate
his elder brother. T. then says the word a second time,
partly in pleasure at his own creative ability, partly because
he is pleased that J. has accepted the word. Then J. repeats
the word. One might think that T's repetition of the word
was perseverative ; but this explanation is not permissible
in the sense which Ach has given to the term, for T. *wants*
to reproduce his creation, it does not reproduce itself.
" The course of a process of consciousness governed by a
determination is *intentional*, i.e. the appearance of the
ideas takes place in harmony with the person undergoing

[1] E. Köhler's statement (p. 54) " that the child can only use the
superlative when it has learnt to count up to three " is probably based on
an unjustifiable assumption of logic in the child's method of thinking.

[2] E. Köhler's Ann, for a reason which cannot be explained linguistically,
called a little celluloid doll " Toti " (p. 45) and a rubber ring on the big
toe of a plaster cast of a foot she called " Pullenisch ".

the experience . . . whilst the appearance of purely perservera-
tive ideas takes place *unintentionally*, i.e. the idea reproduced
is in this case known as present only *after* its appearance "
(Ach, Kühle, Passarge, p. 205). We may only speak of
perseveration here if we understand Ach's theory in the
modification suggested by us. (*e*) The striking construction
" pleased over " instead of " pleased at " was probably
picked up by the children from the servants. (*f*) Because
the book slips and slides on the bed-clothes it is naughty,
but J. is at once sorry for his harsh judgment, which might
offend the book, and so in the same breath he adds that it
is a nice book. Ambivalent estimates of people and things
are met with extremely often in the mentality of the child :
contradictory and contrary properties are at first not
mutually exclusive for the child, as they are for the
harmonized logic of the adult. (*g*) J. takes what his mother
has just read out literally. He does not see the meat shown
in the illustration get covered with water immediately his
mother reads about it. We shall have to refer several
times to J's tendency to take literally everything read
to him.

The above conversation is decidedly governed by its
situation. The verbal utterances are chiefly caused by what
the children see as they turn the pages of the cookery-book.
The conversation is carried on to a much less degree by the
children mutually influencing each other, though this factor
too is not entirely absent.

2

10.10.25. J. comes home from a walk at noon. Before
he takes off his coat he asks for the cookery-book. Opening
it at a page where there is a picture of a dwarf he says :
" The dwarfs must see my sweater, they will laugh."

Discussion.—Here we have only a very brief monologue,
but it seems to us worthy of inclusion. There can be no
doubt that J. is firmly convinced that the dwarfs will be
pleased to see his new sweater, of which he is so proud.

For him " laugh " is synonymous with " be pleased ".
J. treats pictures of men and animals in certain respects
just the same as living beings.

3

13.10.25. The children are playing in bed in the morning.
They are giving each others parts to play.

J. : " I am the baby." (*a*).

M. : " I think you'll always be the baby."

T. : " When Baby grows up he'll still be called Baby." (*b*).

M. : " We'll soon begin to call you both by your names,
shall we Theodor ? "

T. : " But it's sure to get forgotten."

M. : " What shall we call you, Wilhelm Theodor or only
Theodor ? "

T. : " I want to be called Bubi still." (*c*).

M. : " Baby, shall we call you Julius Gregor or Julius
or Gregor ? "

J. : " I want to be Papa and have a motor-bike." (*d*).

M. : " If you want to be Papa then you must have a
Mama too."

J. : " I've got you.

M. : " No, you must have a wife, you know I'm Papa's
wife."

J. : " I don't want a strange wife." (*e*).

T. : " But then she won't be a strange wife."

M. : " Bubi, do you want a wife ? "

T. : " No." (*g*).

Discussion.—Here we have one of the numerous character-
games, which had been very popular with the children for
about a year.[1] At this time the children were often called
by their pet names, but only in the family circle. T. was
called Bubi and J. Baby. In the character-game they are
going to play J. wants to be the little baby, whilst T. has
to play the part of the father (*a*). (*b*) T. fears that the
habit of calling J. by his pet name will not be so easily
dropped—a fear which proved fully justified by the

[1] Cf. D. und R. Katz, *Die Erziehung im vorschulpflichtigen Alter*, p. 74 ff.,
Leipzig, 1925. Quoted as Katz, " Erziehung."

experiences of the next few months—and that, consequently, even when his brother is grown up he will have to go through life as Baby. He feels this pet name to be a disadvantage for his brother much more strongly than with reference to himself. As we see from (c) he does not want to give up his own familiar pet name, Bubi, of which he is probably fond. A few months later when the family had got used to calling him T., he actually felt hurt when an acquaintance who had no knowledge of the change of names addressed him as Bubi. (d) J. has not understood the meaning of the question. When he is given the possibility of being or becoming some one other than Baby, then at once he wishes to be Papa and—have a motor cycle. Papa indeed possesses no such vehicle, but the children have more than once suggested to him that he should buy a car or motor cycle. Here the conversation takes quite another turn ; up to now it has maintained quite well its initial theme of " name changing ". (e) All but those rabid psychoanalysts who delight in discovering the Œdipus complex in conversations as soon as possible will find quite a harmless explanation of J's remark, " I have you," that means, " you love me and I love you, why can't it stay like that always ? " What is meant by " having a wife " is not understood. A " strange " wife is rejected, J. will have nothing to do with such a person. T. discovers quite rightly (f) that a wife with whom one always is cannot any longer be spoken of as " strange ". The fact that T. who has a better conception of the relationship of man and wife also rejects a wife for himself is probably due fundamentally to his own character. T. does not make friends with people as easily as J., who find no difficulty in getting on friendly terms with entire strangers in the street or the tram. In later conversations J. on occasion refers to his " wife and children ".

We consider it necessary to justify our rejection of psychoanalytical methods in the case at issue. T. and J. were not only at the time of the conversation, but even when this book was first published, in the best sense of the word sexually innocent, and that although we have never regaled them with the fairy tale of the stork but from the very first have instructed them about the origin of human beings in a psychologically intelligible way which they could understand. So in a certain sense they are also " sexually enlightened ".[1] In our talks we had touched on the relationship of mother and child, but never on the part played by the father in procreation, for the simple reason that the children had never extended their questions about the origin of people in this direction. We have never noticed any trace of sexual curiosity in our children. Many months later T. declares (Conv. 101) that he can only distinguish boys from girls by the different length of their hair when they are small children who are dressed alike. Men are distinguished from women chiefly by their clothing, it does not seem to have occurred to the children that there are differences in physical make-up. We consider it quite out of the question for the children to have made this discovery and kept it secret from us, because a state of absolute confidence existed between us. The children might distinguish men from women in other ways than by clothing, e.g. by speech and conduct, but these differences lie for them on the same level as those, say, between Europeans and negroes and have nothing at all to do with sex difference in the real sense of the words. For the children this difference simply does not exist.

4

15.10.25. Afternoon. M. is sewing a button on F's coat.
J. : " Mama, what are you doing ? "
M. : " I am sewing a button on."
J. : " Why ? "
M. : " Because Papa has pulled it off."
J. : " When Papa was a little boy ? "

Discussion.—J. simply cannot imagine that even adults sometimes lose buttons from their clothes. That only happens

[1] Cf. the remarks about this subject in Katz, *Erziehung*, p. 107, and the following conversations.

to children, and is indeed a sign of wildness or roughness.
J. is still entirely lacking in temporal orientation, else how
could he think it possible that the suit F. wore as a child
is still in existence ? But perhaps the assumption of such
· powers of thought in the child is intellectualizing the child's
statement too much. Perhaps the child's way of looking
at it is to be considered rather more intuitive :   button
come off, therefore child like me.

5

16.10.25.   Morning.
M. : " Bubi, are you going to water the flowers ? "
T. : " Yes. I say, I think it will grow into a tree."
J. : " Yes, it will grow into a tree."

Discussion.—A very natural supposition of childish
botany, that indoor plants will keep on growing till they
are trees. But what T. only surmises is taken for granted
by J., just because it is said by his elder brother.

6

16.10.25. The children come home from a walk and tell
what they have done.
J. : " I stroked a little dog."
T. : " Baby may stroke *strange* people's dogs only if they
permit him.
E. : " The lady did give permission."
J. : " The lady did give permission."

Discussion.—This short conversation is included for
characterological reasons. Although in training our children
we never did anything which might cause them to be afraid
of, or to have an aversion of, animals of any kind, and on
the contrary tried to arouse in them interest in all living
creatures, yet T. displayed a natural shyness towards
animals. He certainly revealed an unusually strong interest
in them, but he exercised it only from some distance.
Only with an effort did he bring himself to stroke dogs,
rabbits, and other small animals. We consider this due to

conduct based on inborn characteristics, which, however, were additionally motivated by an experience T. had with a monkey in the Zoo when the animal—probably with no malicious intention—seized his sleeve and tugged at it, causing T. to burst out into terrified screams. T. was quickly rescued from this position, but, as we hear from his later remarks, this experience made a deep impression on him. It may have had such after effects as to render more difficult our struggle against his aversion to animals. In complete contrast to T., J. was from the very first at home with all animals and took them in his arms or on his lap. Even those creatures which are sometimes slightly repugnant even to adults, such as salamanders, toads, snails, and earth-worms he would pick up and caress against his cheek, so that we had to wage, with due caution, a struggle in his case against a rather too extensive love of animals. We are sorry to say that at the time of the publication of this book, the constant example provided by T's aversion to dogs is causing J. to be to some extent suggestively influenced in this direction. At the time of recording the above dialogue there was no trace of any aversion, and T. finds it particularly wrong that J. has stroked, above all things, a *strange* dog in the street. As a matter of fact they had been forbidden by us to do this.

7

16.10.25. Afternoon.

M. : " Bubi, do you want to write on your slate ? "

T. : " Yes.   Mama, I want to have a guide-book " (i.e. note-book). (Draws on the slate.) " Mama, I have made a house. Mama, what is this ? "

M. : " A house."

T. : " No, a door. Here is the tower where Malin (a fairy-tale character) lives." (Discovers that he has J's slate.) " This is not my slate, bring the other. Yes, that's mine with the cord. There used to be a sponge there. The cord is broken off." (E. ties on a new cord, wetting it with her tongue). " You don't do it like that."

E. : " Yes you do."

T. : " You dirty dog." (*a*).

M. : " You mustn't say things like that."

T. : " But she was licking it."

M : " You can't get the cord through the hole if you don't."

T. : " To-morrow you must come earlier."

E. : " I can't come earlier, I have to go to school."

T. : " So have I (kindergarten) you cheeky thing." (*b*).

M. : " You must not say that." (The children sit in boxes which represent ships in the character-play they are just starting.)

T. : " Pai." (A word used from the age of two to indicate " leave the room ".)

M. : " Baby, do Pai too."

J. : " I'm the porter." (*c*).

M. : " Well, porter, do Pai."

T. : " I'm the captain."

M. : " And who am I ? "

J. : " You are the woman on the ship." (*d*).

G. : " Who am I ? "

J. : " You are not a woman." (*e*).

M. : " Isn't grandma a woman ? "

J. : " No, of course, she's grandma." (*f*).

Discussion.—(*a*) At times the struggle against the children's bad habits is extremely difficult because of the bad example set by the servants. T. is here blaming an action of E's, which he has been previously told is wrong. It is by no means an edifying situation when as in such cases the child becomes the instructor of the instructor and the parents have the unpleasant task either of belying their own principles by condemning the child's rude remark, or of remaining silent and thereby admitting the truth of the child's statement, with a consequent weakening of the authority of the youthful instructor. The case at issue is this time not very tragic, but we shall find situations where the influence of the instructors has a fatal effect. (*b*) " cheeky thing " (Frechdachs) was just at this time a fashionable slang term, doubtless imported from the kindergarten T. was attending. This slang word had so impressed him that he used to trot it out on every suitable and unsuitable occasion.[1] In the character-play, to which the second part of the conversation refers, J. has at first taken over the part of porter (c) which he expects to be respected by the adults, as well as in all other ways. Each of the parts played by the children was usually kept by them for some length of time. In these character-plays it was quite frequent for other persons present (as here their mother (d) and grandmother) to be included (e). M. is the " woman on the ship ". That a person can or must be a woman if she is his grandmother not only does not appeal to the childish logic, but is even expressly denied. The term " woman " is far too colourless for J., the idea " grandmother ", on the other hand, has an emotional significance to which he was about this time deeply attached.

The first part of this conversation is governed chiefly by the situation and remains so, it develops consequent on the completion of actions of an external nature. The second part develops more from within itself, from a point governed by the character-play.

8

17.10.25. Morning in bed.
J. : " Mama, how does Mr. Krause sleep ? " (a).
M. : " I don't know. I've never visited Mr. Krause in his bedroom."
T. : " Only the doctor can do that." (b).
M. : " Mr. Krause probably sleeps in bed, like anyone else."

Discussion.—(a) It is not easy to say what caused J., in bed early in the morning, to ask about the sleeping conditions of Mr. Krause, our shoemaker, to whom the children used occasionally to take shoes to be repaired. Of course we cannot dispose of the affair by saying that the

---

[1] It is very interesting to note what terms of slang and abuse children use and to discover how they pick them up.

constellation " being in bed " has called forth associatively
the idea " sleep of Mr. Krause ", for numerous other ideas
easily related to this constellation were not reproduced.
We could discover no external stimulus to the reproduction
which did actually take place. For neither in what proceeded
the remark had there been any mention of Mr. Krause or
of things connected with him nor had J. seen any shoes, etc.,
which might have reminded him of a shoemaker. Is it
perhaps a reproduction made possible by unknown associative connecting links ? This question cannot be answered
with certainty for there are no good reasons either for
denying or affirming it. Then the only alternative is to
regard the reproduction as a spontaneous idea ? This
question requires further consideration in the light of the
basic ideas of Ach and his school regarding perseveration.
As they require to be illustrated by examples and dealt with
at some length, it will be better to conclude the discussion
of the conversation before dealing with them. (b) T's statement arises from his experience that the doctor is always
admitted to the bedroom. M. thinks it best to end the
conversation with a reassuring answer to J's question.

Through the researches of Ach, Kühle, and Passarge,
the study of perseveration has been extended in a way
rather important for child psychology. We shall
characterize here the parts important for our work. It is
not only individual ideas which may perseverate but also
feelings and intellectual mental states of the most varied
kinds. Perseveration influences the course of mental processes in children much more strongly than in adolescents
and adults because the other tendencies, associative and
determinative, which play a part in deciding the process,
are not yet so strong. Müller and Pilzecker state that
perseveration tendencies fade away very quickly, but
Passarge, on the contrary, says he has (in favourable
circumstances) discovered them hours and even days
afterwards. Müller and Pilzecker claim that the perseveration tendencies prove effective chiefly when the factors

otherwise impinging on the consciousness are not of particular strength or continuance, whilst Ach believes he has discovered that they are capable of being effective even if the consciousness is occupied by other forces. In this new form the science of the study of perseveration tendencies seems to us of importance for an explanation of the form assumed in many conversations. We assume that perseverations have played a part in guiding the child's conversation in those cases where a child starts a conversation by referring to some matter previously talked about, without connecting it in any way with the present situation and with no introductory statements, and in every case where the child gives a new turn to the conversation by using a former theme without any associative bridge being perceptible. Then we speak of spontaneous former themes of conversation. We do not dismiss the possibility that one or other of the cases mentioned here can also be explained by assuming that the child uses associative by-paths, which would perhaps be discovered if the child could come to our aid with his self observation. But the large majority must nevertheless be explained as perseverations.

We consider that the Ach theory needs modifying in one point in order to be used in explaining the form of our conversations to the extent planned. We feel it necessary to tone down in this theory the contrast made between the intentional and non-intentional appearance of ideas. It may be that the new thought which causes the child to begin a conversation or to give a new turn to one already begun springs up non-intentionally, but as soon as it is uttered and receives verbal form it is taken over already by the child. There is here no clear dividing line. The child's spontaneous ideas are almost without exception interesting or, not to make them too important, amusing thoughts and subjects which the child will take possession of in order to display them to adults. In our conversations we do also come across perseveratively governed turns in the conversations which rather escape from the child than are willed by him, but these are in the minority. In order to distinguish them from the others we shall designate them in the individual discussion as purely perseverative.[1]

J. uses purely perseverative turns of conversation more often than T. They are probably to be considered as a lower stage in the method of carrying on conversation. And on the whole perseveration is much more frequent in the younger boy than in his elder brother. That is fully in agreement with Ach's theory of the decrease of perseveration with increasing age. New perseverations breaking through cause the conversation to leap from one subject to another ; remaining on one theme takes place after a struggle with the numerous other spontaneous themes which break through. How it comes about that in one particular case this theme and not another arises spontaneously cannot usually be determined, and we shall have to make this admission more than once in discussing the formal side of the conversations. Without descending to the teleological methods once so popular in psychology but now justly discredited, we may say that the effectiveness of spontaneous ideas is practical to the extent that it enables the child to inform himself about numerous quite different subjects, even though this takes place at the cost of the deeper dialogue of a conversation remaining on one theme. The theory can only be applied to child psychology if we assume, as Ach does, that the interesting themes are present perseveratively for some time and that they can exert their influence even if the consciousness is otherwise occupied. But our experiences in the conversations found nothing to support Ach's assumption that perseveration is more manifest when children are tired. Our evening conversations, carried on when the children were in a tired state, showed not the slightest increase in turns of conversation governed by perseveration.

[1] What we call " purely perseverative " is akin to what W. Riese terms " iteration," " Über einige motorische Herdsymptome," *Psychologie und Medizin*, vol. 2.

9

18.10.25. Morning in bed. M. has a note-book in order to make brief notes of what the children say. On this day and the next we tried to write down notes in the presence of the children. Although the children never thought of connecting M's writing with their own utterances, yet we gave up this method afterwards. These two days form the only exceptions to what we said previously about the method of recording the conversations.

J. : " Is that paper ? Are you writing a picture ? Show me the picture. To-morrow you must read the picture to us (a). We must keep this or we might lose the picture." (M. turns over the pages.) " Here we'll put a picture. Here we'll put arm-pit, shoulder, elbow (b). What shall we write next ? Arm-pit, shoulder, elbow ? Where is the arm, we have bound it up " (c). (M. points every time to the written word.) " Where is the face ? And where are the eyes ? " (d). (M. turns over the page, to write on the other side). " And what shall we write here ? "

M. : " What would you like ? "

J. : " Arm-pit (Achsel). And where is Axel ? (e). Where is the arm ? " (M. points to the written word.) " And where is the other arm ? And where is the baby ? " (M. turns over the page.) " And what shall we write here ? And where are the eyes ? "

M. : (points to the written word). " Here is ' eyes '."

J. : (points to a line under the word eyes). " That's a hand." (f). (J. places his hand on the paper). " Mama, write my hand." (g). (M. sketches J's hand.) (J. places his thumb on the paper.) " Now write my thumb." (When this is done J. points to his other (bandaged) hand and asks by signs for it to be " written ". Then, with the same request, he places his whole face on the paper).

Discussion.—The conversation is entirely bound and governed by the situation. The questions J. asks are all directly connected with what M. is doing with the note-book. M. purposely exercised a certain restraint, so that J. would express himself freely, and therefore the conversation is almost a monologue. Consequently this conversation is on a lower level than most of those not bound to a situation and where an adult takes part, but on the other hand it gives us an interesting insight into J's attitude towards the problem of writing, the mystery of which always attracts him whenever he sees his parents occupied with it, and which he would like to solve. (*a*) Writing means for J. about the same as representing things in a simplified but comprehensible way. For how can one possibly understand the letter the picture brings, and transform it into something with meaning, if what is to be seen on the paper does not consist of pictures ! And so he thinks it ought to be possible to read out a picture. Pictures can be understood, series of pictures can be interpreted and the black symbols on the paper must have, for the adult at least, the character of pictures.[1] How close the child with his naïve equalization of drawing and writing, of interpretation of picture-language and reading of letter-words approaches here the actual connection between picture and writing given by developmental psychology. Such a category of experience, active on two sides, the one perceptual imagining and the other abstract symbolism, may actually have been known to the eidetic inventor of hieroglyphics and is perhaps even yet known to many civilized peoples like the Chinese whose written characters are closely connected with pictorial writing. The Chinese may perhaps actually see in a man the ideogram for man, all the more so if, as Jaensch suggests, they are by nature inclined to eidetic vision and so bring a strongly subjective component into their perception.[2] Moreover there is every indication that J. experiences vivid images which mislead him often into giving impossible accounts of imaginary experiences, when it can only be imagination or descriptions he has heard from others. Such occurrences, which will be repeated in later conversations, have not been met with at all in T. In all probability,

[1] The child has to learn " that names belong to quite a different reality from things, namely to speech-reality, which is not itself concrete but represents concrete things." (Werner, p. 183).

[2] E. R. Jaensch, *Ueber den Aufbau der Wahrnehmungswelt und ihre Struktur im Jugendalter*, 2nd ed., Leipzig, 1927, 192 f.

T. is non-eidetic, whilst we could probably assume J., with his beaming, sparkling eyes, to belong to Jaensch's so-called B type. This would agree with what we have previously said about J's equalization of writing and drawing and with many other of his subsequent reported utterances. J. always gave the impression of imagining he was experiencing what M. told him was the meaning of the written word, not in a pale colourless form, but as a perceptual embodiment. Moreover, we may mention here that although eidetic phenomena may make a contribution, perhaps of considerable value, to the interpretation of the formal side of the child's world, yet they are less able to contribute to an understanding of the content of this world. Just as the greatest imaginable difference of subjective phenomena in which a logical proposition—for instance, a mathematical theorem—is stated does not in the least effect the essence of this proposition, so also however great the difference in the subjective ideation of a large number of children, from pronounced eidetic to equally non-eidetic types, the form of ideation is quite without bearing on the content. (b) About this time J. had suffered a slight injury to his left collarbone, and the doctor was endeavouring to accelerate the cure by binding up the whole left arm.[1] When winding the bandage round the arm the words, "arm-pit, shoulder, elbow," were always repeated, and greatly amused the children. Why does this sequence of words occur to J. just at this moment? Perhaps because they were perseveratively readier than any others, but the reproductive force of perseveration may have been associatively increased by the fact that the word "put" in the sentence, "Here we'll put a picture," has by association led to the well-known formula, so often used when binding up the arm, "Now we'll put it on arm-pit, shoulder, elbow." Pure perseveration causes the sequence to be repeated at (c) and from this point the ideas easily proceed to the arm. M's action in

[1] Cf. D. und R. Katz, "Verhalten eines Kindes bei Behinderung eines Armes," *Zeitschr. f. Psychol.*, vol. 102, 1926.

pointing each time to the written word can have a confusing effect, although it is only responding to the child's inclination to see the object in the written characters. The conversation assumes to some extent the character of an experiment, but on the other hand it affords valuable data. (*d*) J. expects face and eyes to be added to the part of the body already there. (*e*) The two words Achsel (shoulder) and Axel (a young friend of J's) are the same in sound and trick J. by making him glide associatively from the one to the other and replace one by the other. (*f*) It is possible that J. does actually see a hand in the line on the paper. It may be a crude external similarity which plays its part here : the hand is elongated ; so is the line ; the line becomes the hand, as it were. Once more we get an obvious expression of the close relationship experienced by J. between writing and pictorial representation, for when he has asked for the hand, the thumb, the bandaged arm, and finally the whole face to be " written ", in each case he attempts to transfer something of the particular member to the paper by making contact each time between the member to be " written " and the paper it is to be " written " on.

10

19.10.25. Morning in bed. M. has a note-book.
T. : " Mama, will you give me the little book ? "
M. : " No."
T. : " Do you need it for ever and ever ? Write Bubi Katz." (M. does so.) " Mama, am I older than you ? " (*a*).
M. : " No ; I am older."
T. : " You are bigger. How old is Papa and how old was he on his birthday and how old is Baby ? (*b*). Why do you write so much and always make dots ? (*c*). Mama, may I have some newspapers ? "
M. : " No, I haven't read them yet."
T. : " You are very curious. Read them then." (*d*).
J. : (has not taken part in the conversation, but meanwhile been turning the pages of the cookery-book). " There is a dwarf. Where are the other dwarfs ? There are two dwarfs. And where are the fishes ? Why don't you show me the pictures ? " (*e*).

Discussion.—(*a*) One might perhaps be surprised that T. asks such a question. Does he really not know that he is the younger ? In many subsequent conversations it will be revealed that both children (as indeed all children of this age) display a remarkable helplessness with regard to all details of time and age : however, we feel certain that T. only asks the question whether he is older than his mother because of a momentary lack of thought, and that he would have given the correct answer if he had been asked directly who was the older. (*b*) It is not quite clear how we are to interpret " you are bigger ". Is it " whoever is older is also bigger ", or " older means the same as bigger ? " We incline to the former interpretation. Of course it would have been possible to get information on this point by directly asking the child, but then the conversation would at once have taken on the form of an examination and that was to be avoided as much as possible. From the relation between the ages of M.–F. it is but a step to the question about the ages of the remaining members of the family. F. had had a birthday just previously so that the memory of this emotionally memorable family event made the child desirous of learning the father's age from this definite point of time. Doubtless T. thinks that the birthday which is so much spoken about, exerts in some way a decisive influence on the formation of the age, and that one as it were becomes older *through the birthday*. (*c*) When T. notices that M. is writing, the conversation takes a new turn, but T. has no idea that what his mother is writing has any connection with what he is saying. (*d*) Curious has here the meaning merely of " anxious to get to know things ", and is not a term of reproach. T. only means that his mother is fond of reading in order to find out new things. (*e*) J. meanwhile has not allowed the conversation between M. and T. to disturb his enjoyment of the cookery-book. His utterances and the questions (with the exception of perhaps the last) are to be considered as a monologue of thoughts expressed aloud rather than as remarks addressed to M.

F

II

13.11.25. We had been to the theatre with the children
in the afternoon. The fairy tale " Snow White " had been
performed by a company of dwarfs. The following conversation took place in the evening in bed.

T. : " Why was the hunter so small in front of the
queen ? "

M. : " The hunter was kneeling before the queen and so
he looked so small."

T. : " Were those real trees in the forest ? "

M. : " No, they were painted trees."

T. : " But how could they charm away the house so
quickly (referring to change of scene) (*a*).

M. : " The house was not charmed away.   Workmen
moved it all away."

T. : " But Mama, the stove is made of stone, surely they
can't move that away so quickly (*b*).   Mama, do you know
who the old man (the Lord Chamberlain) was like ?   Just
like Pipo."   (Clown who had been in a children's festival
play in Warnemünde.)   " Do you know how the old man
looked in his looking-glass and the looking-glass said
nothing ? " (*c*).

Discussion.—The children had been highly delighted with
the play, but with this difference, that whereas T. could
follow the course of the action easily, J. was more pleased
by individual episodes such as the appearance of the dwarfs.
(*a*) As the conversation shows, the illusion had been very
strong in T's case ;   he thought he had seen real trees
and a real house, which could only have been changed and
removed by magic.   Well, he thinks, at least the stove must
have been made of stone (*b*) and so could not be so easily
moved away.   (*c*) In the theatre T. had laughed a great deal
at the comic figure of the Lord Chamberlain, and to our
surprise he had completely understood many subtle points
in his behaviour and conversation.   He held his sides with
laughter when the man, aping the queen, peered into his
pocket-mirror and asked it a question, to which the mirror
did not reply.   He rightly grasped the comic element which
the Lord Chamberlain had in common with the clown

seen in Warnemünde four months previously. Here we may make the general remark that both children had a decided sense of humour, which we carefully sought to cultivate and develop. We believe that it is impossible to rate too highly the value of humour as a weapon against the hardships of life, both great and small, and have endeavoured to bring up our children according to this precept. Happy is the man who has chosen humour as his outlook on life.

12

15.11.25. Evening in bed.

T. : " Mama, Auntie O. says I must put my hands under the bedclothes (in bed)."

M. : " Did you tell Auntie O. that you are not allowed to keep your hands under the clothes ? "

T. : " I did tell her, but Auntie O. said, I must keep my hands under the clothes."

Discussion.—This conversation serves as a proof of how injurious can be the effects produced by a badly informed governess, and how she can destroy the child's laboriously acquired good habits. From their earliest days we had accustomed the children to place their hands outside the bedclothes when sleeping, so that they might not be tempted to touch their bodies. This habit did indeed become ingrained in the children, so that they always automatically placed their hands outside the covers or under their heads. When Auntie O. now orders T. to act contrary to his training, and insists on it, even when the child explains that his parents do not allow it, she is not only doing momentary harm, but is undermining her own authority over the child.

13

24.11.25 The day before T. had been naughty. M. had said to him in bed in the evening, " We will pray to-day that you may not be naughty again," to which T. had replied, " It won't be any use." (*a*).

M. : " You must force yourself, you must want to, then you will be able to."

T. : " Not as quickly as all that." (*b*).

In connection with this conversation, the following short dialogue took place the next day.

M. : " To-day *was* better than yesterday."

T. : " It was the day before yesterday.   It was some use." (*c*).

Discussion.—(*a*) T. is at first not convinced of the practicability of a firm resolution in the struggle against his own weaknesses, or at least he does not believe in any speedy effect (*b*). The retrospective consideration of the following day, however, gives him a proof of the efficacy of a good resolution (*c*). The fact that T. is a full twenty-four hours wrong about the time when he was naughty, may not be merely confusion, but due to a desire to push this day which saw his naughtiness farther back into the past.

14

4.12.25.   Evening in bed.

T. : " Mama, the giant Goliath had a stick, didn't he ? He thought his stick was small, but David thought it was big " (*a*).

M. : " Yes, the stick seemed big to David."

T. : " Heidi B. is my best friend, because she is rough and just like a boy."

Discussion.—The story of David and Goliath had interested the children exceptionally. Here, as usually in fairy tales the principle of contrast had its effect.[1] T. and J. were constantly referring to this story as conversation 21, 22, and 25 reveal. It may be said that the giant with his abnormal strength not only aroused greater interest but more sympathy than did David. At this age morals are obviously not esteemed as highly as physical strength and size (*a*). T. has already a sense of the relativity of size. What appears small to the giant appears big to the tiny David. Here the contrast principle is already affecting

---

[1] Ch. Bühler, *Das Märchen und die Phantasie des Kindes*, 2nd ed., Leipzig, 1925.

T's statement, for really he ought to proceed from a stick which appears of normal size to Goliath. But the statement is doubtless a good performance in logic (*b*). The transition of the " best " friend comes without any obvious stages. Perhaps it is governed by the battle atmosphere surrounding the David-Goliath complex, an atmosphere often connected with Heidi. Be that as it may, here the criterion of value for the little friend is noteworthy : she is rough and just like a boy. A little girl in the neighbourhood with whom the children had previously liked to play, was completely rejected as a playmate about this time, because she was too quiet and too phlegmatic. She did not fall in with the boy's boisterous spirits, whilst Heidi would join in wholeheartedly.

15

10.12.25. Morning in bed.

T. (holding a chocolate Father Christmas in his hand) " I'll give you a piece of Father Christmas's face." (T. tries to bite off Father Christmas's face but does not succeed. J. unobserved takes the figure from T's hand and bites the whole head off. T. is pleased rather than vexed about the affair.) " Show me." (J. shows the head and then puts it in his mouth.) " Mama, baby really should have asked me if he might bite off the head " (*a*).

M. : " Yes, he ought really."

T. (gives the whole figure to J.). " Here, you can have all Father Christmas."

M. : " Don't you want him ? "

T. : " No, not without head." (*b*).

Discussion.—This short conversation and the accompanying actions characterize extremely well J's great desire at this time for all kinds of dainties and on the other hand the friendliness and magnanimity of T's treatment of his younger brother. (*a*). Perhaps the logical construction of the modus potentialis is rather unusual in a five-year-old. (*b*). It is a striking fact, that the loss of value as a plaything, when Father Christmas loses his head, causes T. to overlook completely the considerable material loss.

He reveals himself here more as the idealist in contrast to his younger brother, devoted to material pleasures.

16

14.12.25.   Forenoon.
J. (looking at the cookery-book). " Mama, what is that ? "
M. : " That is a swan."
J. : " Is this a cookery-book ? "
M. : " Yes."
J. : " Mama, how does one cook with this book ? " (a).
(Before M. can reply J. goes on.) " What is that, Mama ? "
M. : " That is a piece of meat."
J. : " Meat ? " (softly to himself). Knusperknusper knäuschen (b). (Aloud.) " Mama, who is that, look closely at it, is it a boy or a girl ? "
M. : " It's a dwarf."
T. : " Mama, bad mushrooms are not as dangerous as poisonous ones." (c).
J. : " If you bite a bad mushroom you must throw it away."
M. (reading aloud from the cookery-book, where the word mushroom occurs).
J. : " Where is the mushroom ? " (M. points to the word " mushroom ".)   " I can't see the stalk." (d).

Discussion.—(a) For adults a very amusing question. But really, how does one cook with a book ? M. does not readily find an answer to this unexpected question. (b) Here we have another expression of J's eating complex, which about this period was always on the prowl. From meat he comes associatively to the gingerbread-house in Hansel and Gretel and cannot resist the temptation to utter something connected with it. (c) The distinction between bad and poisonous mushrooms according to their wholesomeness represents a very good achievement in logic, especially as they had never been grouped together by us in this form. We had probably spoken about bad and poisonous mushrooms separately, but the comparison of the two kinds of mushrooms in an independent thought performance by T., is to be designated as a new creation. (d) As mentioned in conversation nine, J. expects a kind of concrete similarity between the objects which are spoken about and the printed word. Perhaps he does really see a mushroom in one of the letters or combinations of letters, but as he says, he cannot see the stalk.

17

15.12.25. Afternoon. T. had had a most unhappy day. He had been very disobedient. Finally F. had had to reprimand him severely, which made him very miserable and he burst into tears. Then F. sat down on the sofa beside him and tried to console him. After some vain attempts he succeeded in allaying his grief and attracting his attention to one of his favourite stories. T. at length listened enthralled, and appeared to have forgotten his trouble entirely.

F. : " Now come with me into the next room and we'll have lunch."

T. : " You think you've consoled me. But it's all no use." (He turned away from F. and remained in this position for some time.)

Discussion.—We include this utterance of T. because it reveals that he had noted the diplomacy in his father's conduct " man merkt die Absicht und man wird verstimmt " ; again it is noteworthy as a proof of the persistence of a mood even at this early age, for it can even break through again when once relief has been afforded.

18

25.12.25. Afternoon.

J. : " Papa, sing the song of the burnt boy." (Vom verbrannten Jungen.)

F. : " What song is that ? "

T. : " My sweetheart has gone away." (Durchgebrannt.)

Discussion.—F. had on a previous occasion sung the first verse of Bierbaum's music-hall song " My sweetheart's gone away " (" Ach mein Schatz ist durchgegangen.") T. was often addressed by F. and M. as " sweetheart " (Schatz) and so for him, " sweetheart " had become

synonymous with " boy ". So " durchgegangener Junge "
(boy run away) became equal to " durchgebrannter Junge "
and then "verbrannter Junge " (burnt boy). F. had no
idea which song J. really meant. But T. was able to solve
the problem obviously because the series of association
causing J's mistake was more familiar to him although he
did not fall a victim to it like his younger brother. But
his sly facial expression clearly indicated that J's mistake
had amused him. He could act as intermediary between
F. and J. because his ideation was turned partly towards
J. and partly towards F.

19

29.12.25.   Evening in bed.
T. : " Why did you stay in Berlin and not go back to
that school ? "   (where M. had previously been a teacher).
M. : " The War came and I couldn't go back again."
T. : " Why couldn't you go back ? "
M. : " The trains were crowded with soldiers and there
was no room for me."
T. : " Wasn't there much to eat then ? " (a).
M. : " No, there wasn't much to eat."
T. : " But Papa had enough to eat, didn't he ? " (b).
M. : " Yes, Papa was a soldier and the soldiers had enough
to eat."
T. : " Why did the soldiers have enough to eat ? "
M. : " If the soldiers had not had enough to eat, they
couldn't have fought."
T. : " And didn't other people have enough to eat ? " (c).
M. : " No, everybody, even the little children, went
hungry."
T. : " Mama, the little babies who hadn't been born yet
were best off, weren't they ? They were lying nice and warm
inside their mamas." (d).
M. : " Yes."
T. : " Mama, when babies crawl out, have they any clothes
on ? " (e).
M. : " No, they are naked."
T. : " Aren't they cold ? " (f).
M. : " No, they're dressed at once."

T. : " Why don't children come out together ? " (g).

M. : " What do you mean ? "

T. : " I mean why didn't I come out together with baby ? " (h).

M. : " That can happen. Then we call the babies twins."

T. : " Of course, they'll have to be smaller then, or else they couldn't very well get out." (j).

Discussion.—(a) From previous conversations T. had probably learned that there was a shortage of food during the war. (b) Two factors play their part here. Firstly the *wish* that Papa *might* have had enough to eat, and secondly the conjecture that soldiers might have been exceptions (T. knew that F. had been a soldier). Why exceptions, he could certainly not have said, as is clear from his next question. (c) The information just gained about the soldiers' food is once again compared with previous facts. (d) A remark in which childish naiveté once again hits the nail on the head. The nourishment of unborn children was actually best provided for ; they got their rations without food tickets. We have previously referred to our attitude towards the question of sexual enlightenment. The answers which M. gives to T's questions (e, f, g, h) reveal our method of enlightening. There is true psychological naturalness about the basic idea from which it proceeds, the intimate, loving relationship between mother and child before birth. In an equally natural way M. answers T's questions about subsequent events. The whole question does not excite the child at all and is treated as an everyday affair. M. does not understand question (g). Of course it does not occur to T. that he would have to be the same age as J. if they had " come out " together ; M. now introduces the idea of twins. (j) T's naive observation once again hits the mark, for often twins are actually smaller than children born singly. T. probably bases his interrogative statement on previous experience that the smaller a thing is the more easily does it come through a hole.

20

1.1.26. Morning in bed.

T. : " Mama, did Papa ever fight the giant Goliath ? " (a).

M. : " No."

T. : " Why didn't Papa fight him ? " (b).

M. : " The giant Goliath was no longer there."

T. : " But Papa did *almost* fight him, didn't he ? " (c). " And Adam and Eve, they were in Paradise, weren't they ? " (d).

M. : " Yes, Paradise was like a great big garden."

T. : " For children, of course ? " (e). " And then Adam and Eve were driven out of there. Where did they go then ? "

M. : " They built a house for themselves and lived in it."

T. : " And then they had children ? "

M. : " Yes."

T. : " And the children ? " (f).

M. : " They had children too."

T. : " And one of these children became God. Mama, is God a man ? " (g).

M. : " No, he's not a man."

T. : " But he was a man. Do you know how I know ? Elli told me all about it. Adam was alone at first and then God created Eve for him, and the serpent could talk. How was that, Mama, animals can't talk, can they ? " (h).

M. : " Well, you know in fairy tales it says that animals can talk."

T. : " Or perhaps God made everything different at first." (j).

M. : " No, I don't think that very much was different in the olden days."

T. : " Mama, it must have been empty in the towns before people were there." (k).

M. : " No, first of all people were there and then these people built the towns."

T. : " How did they do that ? "

M. " First of all they cut down part of the forest and built houses with the trees."

T. : " And here, where Rostock now is, was there a forest here ? " (l).

M. : " Here were large meadows."

T. : " Perhaps the sea was here too." (*m*).

M. : " Yes, first of all the sea was here."

T. : " Was the Teufelskuhle (a large pool near the town walls) there then ? " (*n*).

M. : " Is the Teufelskuhle a brook then ? "

T. : " No, it's a swamp you know, and on Sundays there's always a bowl floating on it." (*o*).

M. : " That's nonsense, there's no bowl floating there No one has ever seen a bowl there. These are stories that only girls tell."

T. : " Why do they tell them ? " (*p*).

M. : " Because they don't know any better ones."

Discussion.—Once again T. has brought up his beloved giant. The question reveals a delightful interpretation of the story which T. has sketched out. Since his father is called David he gives him the honour of having fought a duel with Goliath. When question (*a*) is answered in the negative, question (*b*) follows, still proceeding from the assumption that Papa *did* meet Goliath, that the negative in the first question referred only to a fight. The answer to this second question, that Goliath lived a long time before Papa, does not in the least shake T's unlimited confidence in the desired heroism of his father. Papa " almost " fought with Goliath ; that may mean " if only he had fought him " or it may be regarded as a proof that T. has not grasped the time interval, and believes that Goliath and Papa lived at almost the same time and that Papa almost had the opportunity of fighting the giant. The child's logic does not yet work accurately enough to distinguish clearly between two possibilities ; his logic is still too dependent on his desires, and has not yet freed itself from emotion. (*d*) The transition from Goliath to Adam and Eve is easy to explain, for both these figures belong to the sphere of " Bible Stories ", which stand out among kinds of stories as something apart. (*e*) A big garden can only be intended for children. Then T. returns to Adam and Eve and inquires about the fate of the first human beings after they had been driven out of Paradise.   He has already heard about Cain and Abel and (*f*) tries, with his mother's help, to reconstruct a genealogy of the human race. (*g, h*) Very much against our wishes E. has again been telling the children bible-stories which they could not possibly understand.   We for our part had limited ourselves to those stories, such as David and Goliath, which the children could immediately understand.   Again and again we have discovered to our sorrow how difficult it is to carry through certain fundamental educational principles when the children are coming into contact with uneducated or semi-educated servants, and yet it cannot be prevented.   A short conversation with an uneducated person can cause a confusion in the child's mind, which, due to his great impressionability, it is not easy to remove.   We had decided not to present any religious matter to the children in a form which might sooner or later conflict with their scientific knowledge, for this would only be harmful to true religious education. Even in the question as to whether animals can talk, incomplete as T's scientific experience is, such a conflict is brought up :   animals, therefore serpents also, cannot talk. (*j*) This question is reminiscent of medieval religious discussions. In other conversations too we see a remarkable resemblance to ways of thought which have developed historically in theology, such as those of rational theology (conversation 65).   M. thinks it right to indicate cautiously the immutability of natural laws. (*k*) The idea that empty towns existed first, and that these were then populated by human beings, is suggested to the child from his experience that a house is first built and then people move in ; this experience is then carried over to the whole town. (*l, m*). T. tries to construct for himself a phase of the earth's history.   He himself draws the conclusion that the sea formerly extended to where Rostock now lies.   On the coast at Warnemünde he had noticed how the sea shapes things, and with his own eyes he had witnessed the periodic rise and fall of the tide. (*n, o*).   This question is caused by disturbing impressions due to hearing a blood-curdling story. In the last question (*p*) there is something like a gentle reproach for the girls who tell tales of this sort.

21

2.1.26. Evening in bed.

T. : " Are there really any dwarfs ? " (*a*).

M. : " Why, you were at the theatre yourself and saw Snow White, and there were real dwarfs there."

T. : " I think those were little children, dressed up." (*b*).

M. : " No, they were really dwarfs."

T. : " Where do dwarfs come from then ? " (*c*).

M. : " They are children who are born quite small, and later they don't grow, and stay small, and then we call such people dwarfs."

T. : " Oh, but I'll grow ! " (*d*).

M. : " Yes, you'll grow."

T. : " How can you tell ? " (*e*).

M. : " Your cape is already too small for you, that's because you have grown bigger."

T. : " What did Goliath look like ? "

M. : " I don't quite know."

T. : " And how did he grow into a giant ? " (*f*).

M. : " When he was born he was fairly big, and then kept on growing, so that in time he grew quite big."

T. : " Negroes have white teeth and red tongues, haven't they ? Mama, are there any real negroes or are they only in fairy tales ? " (*g*).

M. : " Yes, negroes are people just like us, only their skin is black."

T. : " But I'm sure they've different habits from us." (*h*).

M. : " What do you mean ? What different habits have negroes ? "

T. : " They show their teeth when they laugh, don't they ? " (*j*).

M. : " Don't we do that ? Just you watch, when we laugh we show all our teeth."

T. : " But they do have other habits. They say ' Hee hee ' when they laugh." (*k*).

M. : " We often say ' hee hee ' too. Negroes are people just like us."

Discussion.—The children had already heard about dwarfs in fairy tales. One day during a walk, F. and T. met a real dwarf of the " small adult " type, with body in almost normal proportions. T. noticed the dwarf before F. and immediately became curious. F. replied, " You see, that is a dwarf." On returning home, T's first thought was to tell M. about this exceedingly impressive experience. He did it in these words, " Mama, we've seen a dwarf, but it wasn't a real one, but a live one " (!). What a strange reversal of the concept of reality ! Up till then the children had only heard of dwarfs in fairy tales, and so the fairy tale dwarf, which the children know in imagination, like all fairy tale characters, is the real one. If a living dwarf meets them, he cannot be a true or genuine one, because the genuine ones are bound up with the fairy tale world of reality. The above incident must be known, in order to understand the starting point of the conversation recorded. Here we have confirmed what we have previously claimed, that the only person who can really understand a child's utterances is one who is thoroughly acquainted with the attitude to things from which they proceed. (*a*) The information that there were really living dwarfs had probably not seemed convincing. The one encountered in the street might of course be an exception, but are living dwarfs quite common in the world ? T. has not yet quite broken away from his old idea that there are only fairy tale dwarfs, and the living ones cannot be genuine. So he will not recognize the dwarf nature of the lilliputians he saw on the stage, although he had been expressly told then that they were not children as he still imagines (*b*), but real dwarfs (*c*). After he has once again been assured that there are living dwarfs, it is quite comprehensible that he should be curious about the origin. (*d*) Here the conversation takes a significant turn. T's remark is less an assertion than a wish, and was uttered with extreme vehemence, which we have tried to indicate by an exclamation mark. What T. would like to express is " I want to grow, I don't want to be as small as a dwarf ".

We are justified in speaking here of " manly protest " in Alfred Adler's term. The child wants to grow big and strong. At present T's life ideal is to grow as big and strong as his father, whereas J. has as it were, an intermediate ideal : he would like first of all to be like his elder brother. This attitude could be proved by innumerable utterances and actions. How justified we are in assuming (d) to be a wish is shown by (e). If T. were quite sure that he will grow and not remain small like a dwarf, he would not need to ask M. for a proof. The cape acts as a very convincing and satisfying proof. (f) Some time ago this transition would have been regarded as a proof of the effectiveness of contrast as an associative principle. The question as to how Goliath became a giant is quite in line with the previous conversation about the origin of dwarfs, but we suspect that behind the question (g) there is hidden something very like a wish, i.e. " How did he become a giant—how can I become a giant ? "—(h) How does T. come to speak about negroes ? Probably from his thoughts about the fairy tale world. Just as dwarfs have occurred only in fairy tales and similar stories, so also must negroes, of which he had never yet seen a living example. T. had only seen them in exaggerated coloured illustrations, and this explains the otherwise incomprehensible remark about teeth and tongues. In reality he says nothing about negroes which might not be equally said of white people. (j) By " other habits " T. probably means " they are considerably different from us ", without being able to specify exactly what this difference is. The remark that negroes show their teeth when laughing (j) is also due to the exaggerated illustrations, as is also the statement that negroes say " hee hee ". Here a strong visual impression finds acoustic expression.

22

3.1.26. Morning. F. is sitting at his writing desk when T. comes over to him and looks attentively at the reading-lamp. Some days previously he had broken F's bedside light.

T. : " When the lamp is broken, the nature of light is not broken as well."

F. : " What is the nature of light ? "

T. : " The daylight."

Discussion.—This short conversation is included because it gives a surprising insight into the child's way of looking at things of a technical-physical nature. From T's statement we learn that he regards the daylight—supposedly the nature of light—as independent of any artificial and destructible source. It is true he does not yet grasp that the sun is the dispenser of daylight, or how the sun performs this task. But from his experience, he knows that the daylight has never yet suddenly failed, like electric or candle light. One may decide for oneself whether a candle or electric light shall give illumination or not, but daylight is different.

23

5.1.26.   Morning in bed.

T. : " Papa, did the giant Goliath always wash in cold water ? " (*a*).

F. : " Yes, that's why he was so strong."

T. : " When did Goliath live ? "

F. : " More than 2,000 years ago."

T. : " Were you living then ? " (*b*).

F. : " No."

T. : " Well how do you know all about Goliath ? " (*c*).

F. : " I read it in books."

T. : " How old are you ? " (*d*).

F. : " I am 41."

T. : " Is that old ? " (*e*).

F. : " No, it's middle-aged."

T. : " What does ' middle-aged ' mean ? " (*f*).

F. : " There are quite young, and quite old people, and in between is called middle-aged."

T. : " Is Elli old ? " (*g*).

F. : " No, she is young.   You know Uncle B. is old and you are young, and I stand just in between."

Discussion.—(a) As we see, interest in Goliath keeps breaking through. We had always impressed on the children the importance of cold water washing for health, and T. easily jumps to the conclusion that Goliath too obtained his imposing attributes by washing in cold water. We consider there is no harm in making use of the child's imagination in order to increase still further his readiness to wash in cold water. (b) The fact that T. considers it possible for F. to have lived 2,000 years ago is another proof of his complete temporal disorientation. In the case of Goliath the existing Goliath-David-Father-David connection causes him to draw false conclusions, this time temporal. (c) A perfectly legitimate question. How can one know about an event which one did not witness ? (d) is the first specific question about F's age. Question (e) probably should be understood as " Do you *call* 41 old " not " Is it really old ". How helpless T. is in face of this concept is shown by question (g), for Elli at the age of 14 makes quite a childish impression.

24

5.1.26. Evening in bed.

J. : " Father Christmas lives in heaven, doesn't he ? " (a).

T. : " Yes, he lives in heaven, he drives very fast in his car, and then the angels come and put a long ladder up to the sky and then Father Christmas climbs up to heaven. (b). Mama, which animal is easiest to catch, is a wild boar easy to catch ? How do they catch them ? " (c).

M. : " They dig a hole, and the hole is covered with branches, and food is put on top. The wild boar wants to get the food and then falls into the pit."

J. : " How are elephants caught ? " (d).

T. : " The elephants are surrounded in a forest, then tame elephants are brought, and then the wild ones go between the tame ones." (e).

J. : " Where do hunters get their guns from ? " (f).

M. : " They buy them at the shop."

T. : " And where does the shop get them from ? " (g).

M. : " From the factory."

T. : " And the factory ? " (h).

M. : " The factory makes the guns."
T. : " What do they make guns of ? " (*j*).
M. : " Of wood."
T. : " But it must be polished." (*k*).
M. : " Yes, the wood is polished and iron is fixed on it."
J. : " How do trees grow ? How do flowers grow ? How do tomatoes grow ? " (*l*).

Discussion.—(*a, b*) The play of imagination around Father Christmas, based on what the children have picked up from stories, and from shop window displays. (*c, d*) The question how wild animals are caught, occupied the children for a long time. They extended their interest to all possible animals one after another, especially to those whose size and fierceness seemed to make their capture particularly difficult. They could listen to stories about catching these animals for hours on end. Their fondness for descriptions of adventure had been aroused. (*e*) T's description is based on an account he had once heard himself, and apparently thoroughly understood. (*f, g, h, j, k*) Here we have a typical case of a whole series of relative questions each of which takes one step backwards towards the genesis of an object. In such cases it is not always easy to find a concluding point. J's questions (*l*) are not directly connected with the original theme, but rather belong to a state of mind produced by the questions " How do such and such things begin ". The " plant " complex is probably prepared by what must be imagined for " forest " (elephants). J's question could not be answered, as he fell asleep literally at the last word.

25

7.1.26. Morning in bed.
T. : " Have we ever had burglars ? "
M. : " No."
T. : " But the door was open once."
M. : " Burglars don't often come."
T. : " Are burglars like other people ? " (*a*).
M. : " Yes, only they are very poor, so they steal bread or something else."

T. : " They ought to play like the hurdy-gurdy man, then they would earn money." (b).

Discussion.—(a) T's knowledge of burglars is probably based exclusively on stories and fairy tales, where of course the act of burglary is greatly looked up to ; for in the family there had been scarcely any mention of burglars. T. has seemingly come to the conclusion that burglars form a distinct category of people, distinguished from ordinary people as negroes or red Indians are from Europeans. T's proposed solution (b) to abolish poverty and thereby the tendency to stealing, shows an inclination to social reform. Remarkable that the child's naïveté once more quite un-suspectingly hits on the truth ; the hurdy-gurdy man is of course a concession to poverty, in order to restrain any tendencies to begging and stealing.

26

10.1.26.   Afternoon, in the electric tram.

T. : " Papa, the elephant is the biggest animal and the mouse is the smallest." (a).

F. : " The mouse isn't the smallest."

T. : " No, the snail." (b).

F. : " There are still smaller ones."

T. : " The flea is of course the smallest." (c).

F. : " No, there are still smaller ones, but you don't know them, they live in the water."

T. : " I know them, but I don't know what they are called." (d).

F. : " How do you know them ? "

T. : " When we were in Copenhagen where the pond is, near the deer, they were in there.   They were quite far away." (e).

Discussion.—T. began this conversation quite spon-taneously in the tram.   Neither the preceding con-versation just ended, nor anything in the present situation, could be cited to make the first remark (a) intelligible. Unless it is the expression of a train of thought which has proceeded to this point by unrecognizable associative paths, we must consider it as a spontaneous, free development. The fact that at this point it is uttered aloud as an interrogative assertion—its obvious form—may be connected with the pleasure felt by the child at contrasting an elephant and a mouse. The series which T. now gives is well worth attention from several points of view. (*b*, *c*) Comparisons in imagination between two objects offered, have frequently been used as intelligence tests.[1] It is seen that T. succeeds in comparing in size, objects selected by himself, from the point of view " the next member must be smaller ". The jump from mouse to flea is not immediately possible ; he requires the intermediate stage " snail " before he can present the flea as the smallest. It may be that T. has actually never yet met a creature smaller than a flea (for the sake of the reputation of his family, " met " is of course not used here in the physical sense : he must have learned of the existence of fleas from stories) or perhaps he would not notice anything smaller than a flea. Whatever the cause, T's further statement that he does however know smaller ones, is very surprising, surprising too in the way it is formulated (*d*). The statement that he knows something but has no verbal term for it, is an exceedingly good intellectual achievement for a child of T's age. But the content of the statement, which is enlarged on by (*e*) is somewhat obscure in meaning. In the pond mentioned by T. there were some frogs, which could be heard as we and the children were walking past. We could not see the frogs, but the children were told that the croaking proceeded from frogs. It is very improbable that T. meant frogs by his mention of the smallest animals, which were a long way off, because he has often seen frogs and even played with them. He must have imagined then some other creatures in the water, or, as is more probable, he does so now, when he is told that the smallest creatures live in water. He has remembered his

---

[1] O. Bobertag, " Ueber Intelligenzprüfungen (nach der Methode von Binet und Simon)," *Zeitschr. f. angew. Psychol.*, vol. 5, 1911, p. 163 ff.

impression of that pond, which the accompanying circumstances must have made memorable, indeed almost legendary to the children. The " quite far away " reproduces that nebulous emotional atmosphere suitable to include even the smallest (purest, frailest) animals.

We should like to direct attention once more to the series followed by T. in this conversation ; mouse, snail, flea linked together, and in the opposite direction we can add the elephant as the largest animal. Such formations of series—this one is from the point of view of size—are of the greatest importance for a study of human thinking in general, and so also for a study of child's thought and development. If three members of a series are given, in most cases we have sufficient data to deduce the law governing the series. Then one proceeds from them to other perceptible members of the series, and even to those which, as border-line cases, are no longer perceptible in the same sense. The developing of all ideals, whether moral, æsthetic or logical, may be based on the natural capacity of man to develop such series. Ideals are rendered possible by transitions from fragments of series which allow the whole law of the series to be deduced. Naturally the law of the series cannot always be formulated mathematically. In elementary mathematics, the transition from the regular polygon to the circle is performed by means of a series of n-angles, where n constantly increases. If the student had not the capacity to grasp the sense of the progress from the perceptually given members of the series, then the transition to $n = \infty$ which is not given perceptually, would remain incomprehensible to him. Series tests of the most varied types are used to determine the intellectual maturity of children ; we consider these tests to be among the most interesting provided by investigations into ability.[1] The investigation into performances when faced by those tasks promises still more valuable information

[1] Cf. O. Bobertag and E. Hylla : *Begabungsprüfung für den Übergang von der Grundschule zu weiterführenden Schulen*. Langensalza, 1925.

about the *a priori* or (to use an expression less hampered by historical connections) formation-law (bildungsgesetzlich) elements in the thinking of children. The formation of series, even though not a strictly mathematical one, shows us T. constructing a series in order to arrange animals according to their size. We may mention here that many Montessori exercises are intended to, and indeed actually do, assist the development of series concepts. This reveals quite clearly that the point of view of totality takes precedence over the atomistic spirit which many Montessori exercises seem to breathe.[1]

27

10.1.26. Evening at the supper-table. The children are ready for bed and have come to say good-night, T. a little before J. F. had the idea of trying an experiment with J. to see how he would react if the identity of his brother were disputed. The following conversation therefore is definitely experimental in character.

J. : " Theo, where are you ? "
F. : (jokingly)." Theo isn't here. (Pointing to T.) That is a little boy who looks like Theo."
J. : " No, it's Theo." (a).
F. : " How do you know it's Theo ? "
J. : " By the colour of his shirt." (b).
F. : " But it's not Theo, only Theo's shirt."
J. : " Yes, it is Theo." (c).
F. : " Look closely at him."
J. : (looks closely at T., who, as is clear from his behaviour, has entered into the joke). " Of course it's Theo." (d).
F. : " How do you know ? "
J. : " By his black eyes." (e).
F. : " But other boys have black eyes too."
J. : " It is Theo though." (f).
T. : " I'm Wilhelm." (g).
J. : (almost in tears). " It is Theo." (h).
F. : " He's going to sleep in Theo's bed."

---

[1] Cf. the corresponding remarks of K. Gerhards : *Zur Beurteilung der Montessori-Pädagogik.* Die Erziehung, 1927.

J. : (bursts out) " You've telled a lie. You know it's Theo " (tries to strike F.).

M. : (consolingly) " Yes it's Wilhelm Theodor, we've only been having a joke."

Discussion.—(*a*) The dispute about T's identity is first of all taken as a joke. (*b*) The attempt to identify T. by the colour of his shirt appears to be beginning with the most external criteria. One cannot consider J's method of proving his brother's identity as explained by merely pointing out that for children, clothes belong much more intimately to their wearer than they do for adults, and so can be brought forward as sufficient proof.[1] We must also attempt to understand why J. does not at once proceed to other seemingly much more obvious criteria. First : how would an adult behave in similar circumstances ? If the identity of the person best known to us were disputed as in J's case, then, according to the circumstances we should only smile at the attempt, or refuse to have anything to do with such foolishness. But how should we behave if the identity was still disputed in all seriousness, the person concerned also adding his denial (just as T. does in our comedy) and speaking of the existence of a double or a twin to such purpose that we became convinced that it really was not a silly joke ? We should look very carefully at the person, study his features firstly in general and then for particularities such as birthmarks, scars, irregularity of teeth or any distinguishing things, which in all probability would not be present in a different person. In any case we should base our decision on these characteristic features which seemed to us fixed, and not likely ever to change. In the case of a living person, clothing is probably the last thing on which we

---

[1] A Kaffir child strikes a person's clothes in order to harm that person ; if it is a child whose clothes are struck, then it may cry out. E. Franke : *Die geistige Entwicklung der Negerkinder. Beiträge zur Kultur-und Universalgeschichte.* Herausg. von Lamprecht Heft 35, Leipzig, 1915.— Our children too were by no means unmoved if their clothes were struck in jest.

should base our identification. If we were permitted to converse with the disputed person, then a totally new series of criteria would be given to us and we should be able to use these new aids. Then, on the basis of these various considerations (because all our expectations about facial characteristics, etc., were realized), either we should make our decision that it is indeed the person supposed, or we should come to the disturbing conclusion that we really had a double before us. But how is the child's effort at identification carried out ? Answer (b) shows that J. is not yet able to distinguish between essential and non-essential characteristics, and so does not start from an examination of the person's features, but takes first the shirt as proof. This does not imply that T's features have been entirely neglected, but only that J. does not base his proof on them first of all. When identity is again disputed, J. does not proceed systematically, but only persists in asserting (c) T's identity, in the hope that the auto-suggestion of his own expression will paralyse the suggestion proceeding from the adults. Only when he is specially told does he begin a detailed examination of the disputed person (d), and base his conclusion on a definite characteristic, the black eyes.[1] (e)   This is to be expected, for the eyes probably take a very important place in a person's face. When the reliability of this criterion is disputed, J. does not fall back on other criteria, but hopes by continued repetition of his conviction (f) to assure the identity. The thing becomes really serious for the little fellow when T. takes part in the cruel play and denies his own identity (g). And how skilfully he does it ! " I am Wilhelm " is not untrue, for T. does possess this second name, but he knows quite well that J. will never remember in his excitement that his brother is called Wilhelm Theodor. Here we have a case of identity disputed even by the bearer of the name, and the name for the child, just as for primitive man,

[1] In reality T. has brown eyes. They were probably called black through affective exaggeration, which is quite frequent in children.

represents an essential element of the person.[1] T's attitude destroys J's equilibrium, he is almost in tears and limits himself to a renewed assertion that it is T. (*f*). But when it is hinted at, that the boy who is not his beloved brother may possibly sleep in T's bed, he breaks down completely. Helpless he tries to relieve his feelings and diminish his grief by attacking his father. The form " telled " (gelügt) betrays clearly the excitement he is labouring under, for such a wrong form would otherwise never occur at his age. Excitement as we see here has exactly the same effect as illness, where the children sink back to a previous lower stage of behaviour, and later acquirements are ineffective. We may add that the united efforts of the parents soon succeeded in calming J., and quite consoled, he retired with T. We scarcely need say that " test " conversations of this kind, cause the child many painful moments and are only permissible as rare exceptions. There are no further conversations of this character recorded.

28

14.1.26.   Morning in bed.
J. : " Mama, God isn't a human being, is he ? " (*a*).
M. : " No.   God isn't a human being."
J. : " There isn't any God, people have never seen God. I know there's no God." (*b*).

Discussion.—(*a*) J. had on occasion heard one of us say that God was not human, and now he is simply reproducing that statement.   Then he twice (*b*) questions the existence of God, and this is clearly a case of making his previous information concrete.   So from " God can't be seen " we get " People can't (and haven't) seen God " and from this he draws the conclusion that God does not exist, since for

---

[1] A friend of mine, an occultist with an extensive practice amongst the native population of Cairo, relates that very often a patient gives a false name, in order to prevent the European doctor from carrying on any magic with his real name, which forms an essential part of his personality. In such cases the doctor used to warn his patients to make quite sure of the fictitious name for purposes of reference in his case-book.—D. Katz.

him only visible things exist. It is extremely difficult to keep children from crudely anthropomorphic concepts in religious affairs. The metaphysical content of religion is always in danger of being misunderstood by children, and it is much easier to explain the other root of religious life, the ethical, in a form which children can understand. Those of our conversations which aim at investigating conscience give evidence of our method of procedure in such matters.

29

15.1.26. Evening in bed.

T. : " When I grow up I'm going to be a sailor and I shall tell my children all about what I see." (*a*).

J. : " When I grow up I'm going to be an engine-driver and I shall tell my children all about the trains." (*b*).

M. : " Oh, so when you grow up you're going to tell the trains about the children." (Loud laughter.)

Discussion.—(*a*) The first (recorded) conversation in which the children speak about their future career. It is natural that every child growing up on the coast will at some time see the sailor's life as his ideal future. As we shall see, this desire of T's is not very long-lived, and is followed by very many others. (*b*) J's wish to be an engine-driver does not last very long either. Really he is here quickly improvising a profession in which he too, like T., his pattern and guide, will have the opportunity of travelling about the world and of telling his children of his adventures. He does not want to be behind his brother in this respect. Both children thoroughly understand and appreciate their mother's joking inversion of trains and children.

30

16.1.26. Evening in bed.

T. : " Mama, how can people tell which animals lived a long time ago ? " (*a*).

M. : " When holes are being dug, sometimes remains of animals are found. From these remains we can discover what animals lived a long time ago."

T. : " Then it can be seen that they were like sheep or perhaps other animals (*b*). Are whole horses found too ? " (*c*).

M. : " Yes, whole horses are found."

T. : " And elephants too ? " (*d*).

M. : " Yes, elephants too."

J. : " Where is meat found ? " (*e*).

M. : " Meat is found everywhere where animals are."

J. : " And where is straw found ? " (*f*).

M. : " In barns."

J. : " How does straw grow ? " (*g*).

M. : " In the fields. On the way to Warnemünde you know there are fields where corn is growing. From this corn we get straw."

J. : " Does straw grow in meadows too ? " (*h*).

M. : " No, grass grows in meadows."

J. : " No, I've seen straw growing in meadows (*j*). Mama, how are lions caught ? " (*k*).

T. : " Big lions can't be caught, but only small ones." (*l*).

J. : " And how are negroes caught ? " (*m*).

M. : " Negroes are people like us, they aren't caught."

J. : " Mama, are there any real crocodiles ? " (*n*).

M. : " Yes, there are real crocodiles."

J. : " But there aren't any musicians, are there ? " (*o*).

M. : " There are musicians too."

J. : " It is telling a lie if people say they have seen a deer, and they say it was a tiger, isn't it ? " (*p*).

M. : " Yes."

Discussion.—(*a*) T. had been interested for some time in the origin of animals. The answer given by M. was too abstract for him. It is characteristic that he at once makes it more intelligible by making it concrete and (*b*) exemplifying it by means of the special case of the sheep, and then immediately generalizes it by adding " or perhaps other animals ". (*c, d*) Whilst sheep were only taken at random as examples of animals, the questions about horses and elephants are asked from a particulary lively interest in these creatures. (*e, f, g*) Whereas T. has asked his questions from a purely theoretical, almost scientific point of view, J's first question, in its form governed by his brother's models, is directed to much more practical affairs, to his favourite meat. And the two succeeding questions about natural products show that J's approach to the question of the development of organic life is from quite a different angle from T. (j) J. proves unteachable and persists in his assertion, not yet distinguishing between meadows and fields. (k) The transition to the lion takes place quite spontaneously (sprunghaft). Really all animals are always prowling about, ready to spring perseveratively into the conversation at any moment. T. proceeds to play a part in informing his brother, using knowledge gained from stories heard previously. (m) It is not difficult to understand the transition from catching lions to catching negroes if it is remembered that negroes are often depicted as wild men and savages. (n) Crocodiles had often been mentioned in the same connection as negroes, so the transition takes place by association. But J. has only heard about crocodiles in stories, and has never met a real one, so he is justified in asking if such creatures really exist. The step from crocodiles to musicians is obviously due to Geibel's song, "A merry musician once marched by the Nile" ("Ein lustiger Musikante marschierte einst am Nil") which F. had often sung to the children, to their great delight. Now it appears (o) that J. has not understood the song, or at least has not understood what a musician is, for he doubts their very existence. (p) The transition is not very obvious. "Telling a lie" might be governed by the thought: "whoever talks of musicians is telling a lie; but why is the lie exemplified by the sentence used here? It is clear what J. wishes to express, but he does not succeed in mastering the correct language to represent it; it should run: it is telling a lie if people say they saw a deer and it was only a tiger.

31

30.1.26.   Morning in bed.
J. : "There aren't any girls on wheels, and if people say there are, they are telling lies." (a).

T. : " Mama, it's so funny to me, how do the things (parcels) get into the mail-vans ? " (b).

M. : " The postman puts the parcels which arrive by train into the vans."

T. : " Now I know, the mail-van drives about the streets and delivers the parcels." (c).

Discussion.—(a) We cannot say how J. came to the construction of this lie. He does not expect an answer to his statement, as his tone of voice clearly reveals the apodictive nature of the sentence. (b, c) Probably when T. was in the street it suddenly struck him as strange that parcels should be found in mail-vans. He has thought deeply about the matter, but could find no explanation, and now places the question before his mother. But why just at this moment ? Perhaps because J's mention of wheels has furnished the bridge to the mail-van.

32

27.1.26. Evening in bed.

J. : " Mama, is God a human being ? " (a).

M. : " No, God is not a human being."

T. : " Is God a bird ? " (b).[1]

M. : " No, God is not a bird."

T. : " Mama, were there any animals before people were living on the earth ? " (c).

M. : " Yes."

T. : " Why didn't the people come first ? " (d).

M. : " It just was so, one can't ask why."

T. : " How shall I ask then ? " (e). " Mama, did the Jews live before God ? " (f).

M. : " No, the Jews knew about God too."

T. : " Are there two Gods then ? " (g).

M. : " No, there is only one God."

T. : " And Auntie O. said that the Jews lived before God." (h).

[1] " When the bell was tolling in the twilight, my mother spoke to me about God and taught me to pray. I asked : What is God ? is he a man ? and she replied : No, God is a spirit ! The church roof faded slowly away amidst grey shadows, the light climbed up the little steeple till at last it sparkled only on the golden weathercock, and one evening I found myself suddenly full of the definite belief that this cock was God." Gottfried Keller, *Der grüne Heinrich.*

Discussion.—(*a*, *b*, *f*, *g*, *h*) All these questions confirm our previous statements (Conv. 30) about the difficulty of giving children an intelligible idea of the metaphysical content of religious matters, and they seem to us to contain a hint to be cautious in one's statements. Question (*d*) is quite justified in the scientific sense, once question (*c*) has been answered in the affirmative. Why should not men have lived before animals? (*e*) T. does not understand M's attempt to explain to him that questions must come to an end somewhere, and that a scientific fact must be accepted as such. T. thinks he has asked in the wrong way and inquires how one must ask correctly in order to get an answer.

33

28.1.26 evening in bed.

T. : " Do animals come to an end too (i.e. do animals die) ? " (*a*).

M. : " Yes, animals come to an end too. Everything that lives comes to an end.

T. : " I don't want to come to an end, I should like to live longer than everybody on the earth." (*b*).

M. : " You need never die, you can live for ever."

Discussion.—We have tried as far as possible to keep away from the children any conception of death, especially in connection with human beings. Of what use would it have been to disturb them with thoughts about death, which must necessarily be extremely mysterious and terrible to them if they hear of it, and yet have no consolation of any kind to support them. Why show these young beings the end of a journey they are only just beginning to make in full and confident vigour ? But once again an unsolicited helper must have interfered in our plans and found it right and proper to tell T. about death, otherwise question (*a*) would never have occurred to him. When his mother gives him a truthful answer, T. for the first time reveals fear of death ; he expresses the will to live by saying in (*b*) that he wants at least longer than anyone else. In view of his distress, M. decides to console the child in the final sentence.

34

2.2.26. Morning in bed.

T. : " Papa, I dreamt last night I was crossing the street with Elli, and when we had turned the corner the moon fell down and rolled across the street. But not the full moon, only the half moon." (*a*).

F. : " That was fine, I should think."

T. : " Papa, once when I was really walking in the street with Auntie O., I saw a Sternschmuck (i.e. star-decoration)." (*b*).

F. : " I think you mean a Sternschnuppe (shooting-star)."

T. : " Yes. Papa, why is there no shooting-moon ? " (*c*). " Where do shooting-stars come from ? Surely it's not the whole star ? A whole star can't fall down, can it ? " (*d*).

F. : " No, it's always a piece of the star that breaks off."

T. : " Papa, Appelschnut is much older than I, she goes now to the proper school. She wants to pull the sun out of the water, isn't that silly ." (*e*).

Discussion.—(*a*) The first account of a dream, not only in these conversations, but the first T. ever mentioned. Both the spontaneity of the account and the content, of thoroughly plausible dream-structure, vouch for the genuineness of the dream and exclude the possibility of invention. It is quite feasible that in a child's dream half the moon should fall down and roll across the street. The reproduction —assuming that the dream is genuine—reveals a good capacity for observing series of experience. A further proof that the dream was genuine is given by the report of an astronomical observation actually made by T. himself (the shooting-star), that is as a sort of contrast to the dream experience. The formation " Sternschmuck " (star-decoration) is a charming invention. Was it produced because decorations are frequently star shaped, or (if we assume a higher performance possible by the child) is it the conception of the shooting star as a firework, as star-decorations ? Perhaps both. (c) Why should there not be any shooting-moons ? Before the answer can be given, T. asks the second question, about the origin of shooting-stars, and gives the answer in question (d), where he states that it is probably a part of the star. The last statement (e) is intimately connected with the preceding remarks. From stars and moon it is but a step to other celestial bodies. Appelschnut is really a living person to T. and not a story-book character. T. here criticizes Appelschnut's intelligence for thinking she can pick up the sun's reflection in water, even though she is now attending school. Poor Appelschnut and poor Otto Ernst, who has represented his heroine as so naïve !

35

12.2.26. Whilst playing in the afternoon.
M. : " Now I'll growl like a bear " (does so).
J. : (screams and weeps).
M. : " Why are you crying ? "
J. : " Oh, I thought you'd bewitched yourself." (a).
T. comes into the room. M. growls again. J. runs away and hides.
T. : (anxiously) " I was a bit afraid you know." (b).

Discussion.—(a) We have no reason to doubt that J. is not pretending to be afraid, but is really very scared that his mother has turned into a bear and is growling. For J. the game had lost its playful character and had become deadly serious, as his cries and tears reveal. How strange : a child who a moment before has seen and been playing with his mother, as his mother, suddenly turns away from her terrified, without her having even been out of his sight or changed her exterior in any way ; he runs away from her when she says she will growl like a bear and utters a kind of bear growl. J. thinks his mother has bewitched herself. What has happened here ? Does J. no longer recognize his mother's familiar well-loved face, and does he under the suggestive influence of ear and eye see in her an animal ? The most obvious parallel is the frequently investigated case of childish play-illusion, in which the child is able to see various objects, e.g. a man, then an engine, then again a house, etc., in the wooden bricks of his building outfit. The child is able to treat the block of wood at one moment as a certain object and the next moment as another object quite different. But whatever may be one's attitude theoretically to the interpretation of the nature of these experiences, they are different from those recorded here in two ways. Firstly, through the strength of the " illusion " and secondly, a fundamental difference, that this is not a case of a play experience, but of an experience which is terribly serious to the child. The interpretation used to explain the illusion-games will therefore not be adequate in this case. Let us ask first of all : is the experience thoroughly serious to J., i.e. does he behave towards his mother in exactly the same way as he would behave if a real bear suddenly came into the room at his mother's request and began to growl ? We must answer this question in the negative : if a real bear came, J. would be much more terrified than he now is. So then his excited conduct towards his mother is not really serious ? Our reply is, he is serious to the same extent as primitive man is serious when he says a man is identical with a snake, a kangaroo or a frigate bird.[1] According to the principle of mystical participation a person can be a human being and animal at one and the same time. And so J. experienced his mother both as mother and as something bear-like. The part played by magical thinking in the child's mental life here appears most clearly, and J. himself speaks in a most revealing way by saying M. has bewitched herself. The law of the identity of persons does not yet apply strictly in the case of the affective thinking of children of this age, there is no contradiction in the fact of a person being a human being and an animal at the same time. For us adults this law of the identity

[1] Werner, p. 222.

of persons may lapse in dreams or delirium. Let anyone try to describe or re-experience when awake what he felt when dreaming about the mingling of two persons or of a person and an animal into one being and he will not succeed, although he never doubts that he really did have the experience. Probably our dream condition corresponds to the state of the emotional waking consciousness of the child. It is impossible for an adult with the resources of normal waking consciousness to live through the experience which J. had. But we can have an empathy, even if only a theoretical one, about our own dream experiences. We can have no doubt of the *possibility* of experiences in which there is a magical element, for they are guaranteed by experiences and also by numerous descriptions in ethnology.[1] How does M. get this magical participation in the quality of being a bear ? By the suggestion given by the word and the mimic-acoustic behaviour, the word probably being more effective. If one simply growls like a bear, without saying anything, the child is probably inclined to laugh, but if one adds " now I'll growl like a bear " it has a decisive irresistible effect. The child succumbs to the magical effect of the word. How often in the history of mankind has something like a mystical power proceeded from words and this power is still active in the child. What is to be our view about the action of the word ? Does it go beyond the imaginative image and *must* it go beyond the visual imaginative image of the thing or person represented ? It is our belief that it is to a great extent independent of the presence of a visual imaginative image in the real sense of the word, and therefore, for instance, acts on the word independent of the eidetic disposition of the child. We do not consider that the fundamental elements of the present case can be explained by reference to J's presumably

---

[1] We mention a few examples. The Bororos maintain that they are Araras (parrots). When dancing many Red Indians identify themselves with the animals whose masks they are wearing, e.g. buffalo, etc. The Huitscholes consider deer and stars to be identical.

existent eidetic disposition. It is by no means necessary that the idea of a bear, of hallucinatory strength, should appear in J's mind at the moment when M. announces that she is going to growl like a bear. The mere presence of such an idea would not explain J's conduct in the least, for it would not need to be at all different from the idea which might be caused during play by the word bear, when it would not be terrifying. The essential point is, that the whole danger-complex connected with the idea " bear ", however that may be represented, is given emotionally. This complex can be conveyed to the senses in various ways, and it is probably transmitted in J's case quite differently from T. whom we suppose to be non-eidetic. But, as we see from (b), T. is also frightened by M's behaviour, although seemingly not to the same extent as J. According to our view this is simply because he is older and not so susceptible to the suggestive force of word and action. If we were to say that it is because as an older child he is not eidetic to the same extent as J., then quite apart from all other factors, we should have to bear the onus of proof that the eidetic state of mind is stronger in earlier childhood, and then gradually decreases—a statement for which as yet there is not the slightest evidence. So for the present we maintain our assertion that there are only slight connections, if indeed any at all, between the eidetic state of mind and the behaviour of the child as we observe it here.[1]

We are able to report similar behaviour by two other children, thanks to the information afforded by a lady of our acquaintance. When this lady plays " Barnstorf " (Zoo) with her two children, aged 2 and 3 years, and growls behind a chair placed as a " cage " the children are afraid and call out " Be mummy again ". The lady thought this was

[1] " Our children are Hänsel and Gretel, Snow-White and the Queen, but Wolf and Grandmother as well, and really think they are the wolf, so that they begin to weep at the exciting points—from fear, for their brother at these moments is really and truly the wolf." Ebel," Die Anfänge des kindlichen Märchenverständnisses," *Vierteljahrsschrift für wissenschaftliche Pädagogik*, 1925, No. 1.

due to a particularly lively sense of fear in her two children,
but this cannot be so, for our children, whom we cannot by
any means call timid, behaved exactly the same in similar
situations.   Once again we see how necessary it is to be
extremely careful in giving absolute verdicts about a child's
performances and behaviour, when there are no facilities
available for controlling the comparisons.

36

12.2.26. Afternoon. T. has dressed up as a Wandervogel
and comes into the room.

M. : " Who are you ? "

T. : " I'm a leader of the Wandervogel." (*a*).

M. : " What is this ? " (a box which T. has hanging on
a cord).

T. : " I put my pipe (Piepe) in that when I want to
smoke." (*b*).

M. : " But don't you know my dear Leader, that you
don't smoke if you belong to the Wandervogel ? "

T. : " But I'm a leader." (*c*).

M. : " Then you ought not to smoke in order to set a
good example."

T. : " I haven't any children to lead yet." (*d*).

M. : " I will recommend some children for you to lead.
What is your name ? "

T. : " Mr. Herzlob." (*e*).

M. : " Have you any brothers and sisters ? "

T. : " Yes, two." (*f*).

M. : " What do they do ? "

T. : " One is a carter, the other a railwayman." (*g*).

M. : " Where is the brother who is a carter ? "

T. : " He works for the cleansing department.   But he
isn't very busy, he has to work very hard." (*h*).

M. : " So your brother works for the cleansing department.
And has the brother who is a railwayman to work hard
too ? "

T. : " Yes, he has to drive a great deal." (*j*).

Discussion.—Several times recently a Wandervogel leader
had visited us, and had aroused the admiration of both
children by his unfamiliar costume.   They showed not only

the usual happy curiosity aroused by strangeness, but also were attracted by the youth and freshness of his appearance. The after effects of the meeting are shown by the disguise T. now adopts. He is not satisfied to be a Wandervogel but has promoted himself immediately to leader (*a*). The part he is playing is then carried on quite logically, and with surprising originality in the invention and adornment of individual details. This is seen at once in the mention of the pipe (*b*), and we may call attention to the use of the Low German word " Piepe " which sounds to the boy more suited to the spirit of the masquerade than the High German " Pfeife " which he knows equally well and would normally use. Although T. can scarcely have heard that the Wandervogel are forbidden to smoke, yet he shows at once complete understanding of the ban and claims for himself a privileged position as leader (*c*). And very skilfully he tries to evade the obligation to set a good example, imposed by his position as leader, by saying that as yet he has no children to lead (*d*). The name Herzlob (*e*) is apparently invented on the spur of the moment, in any case we have never heard him mention the name before, and it must be considered a new creation most suitable for the name of someone acting as a leader of children. At all times T's imagination is quickened by the stimulating influence of dressing up and conversation, in an adult we should class similar behaviour as a moment of happy inspiration. That he has two brothers (*f*) is also a flash of inspiration, and having confessed to this he is compelled on the spur of the moment to invent suitable occupations for them (*g*). Statement (*h*) contains a contradiction, as T. says that his brother in the cleansing department is not very busy and yet has to work very hard. This is the only place in the whole conversation where T. gets into confusion ; here he is obviously led astray by phrases he has taken over from adult conversation without thinking about them. And even his mistake is not very serious, for such an illogicality could also occur in an uneducated person's conversation without being very obvious. The last answer is again quite sensible, and the question is not merely affirmed, but gets a little colouring, with reference to the fictitious occupation of the second brother.

We mentioned that T's ready invention in the course of this conversation reveals that the time was favourable. In general we may say that there are great fluctuations in the children's performances, fluctuations connected with the time of day, the momentary state of health, and also with other inner states of the child's mental life, which cannot be immediately explained. We have already mentioned T's greater tendency to mistakes when suffering from a sore throat ; illness causes intellectual exhaustion, and as our note-book shows, this is so obvious in children in their second year, that a feverish cold can produce a relapse into a period of development passed through several months previously.

37

17.2.26. Morning.

J. : " I should like to be a mail-van driver and a waiter and a tram-conductor." (a).

T. : " On Sundays you'd like to be a conductor." (b).

J. : " And when the calendar leaves are black." (c).

M. : " Then you will be a mail-driver and bring a parcel. Then I'll take you on my lap and give you a piece of sugar and say to you that you are a dear little fellow."

J. : " I want to be a big fellow." (d).

T. : " You are a little shrimp." (e).

J. : " I won't give you any sugar (f). (Turning to M.) I want to be as big as you and I, about in the middle (g). Why wasn't Uncle X called Zitterer ? (J. had heard that this uncle had been nicknamed Zitterbock as a boy.) A goat is an animal and Uncle X is a human being of course, and a goat is only a sheep with horns (h).

Discussion.—(a) Here we get J. mentioning three future professions at once. For some time van-driver and tram-conductor had been the occupations which excited the children's imagination. It is not so easy to say how J.

arrived at his choice of waiter ; perhaps it is the memory of a most impressive waiter in a railway dining-car, seen some months previously. (*b*) Why does T. suggest the conductor's job for Sundays ? Perhaps because Sunday is the busiest day for traffic, and most people are travelling on the trams. (*c*) In the nursery there hung a big tear-off calendar, which the children loved to attend to. The Sundays were distinguished by being printed in red type, and so a red leaf meant Sunday to the children. Often in the nursery we spoke of the " day with the red calendar leaf " instead of Sunday. The term " Sunday " is used much more often than " week-day " and so it is easy to understand that J. uses the visual image " when the calendar leaf is black " to designate the week-days for which he as yet lacks a term. (*d*) A powerful outburst of manly protest ! (see conv. 21). It does not suit his purpose to be called a " dear little fellow ", he wants to be a big fellow. And then T. is tactless enough to point out that he is only a little shrimp (*e*), whereupon J. takes revenge by not giving him any of the sugar (*f*) which he will get some day as a mail-van driver. At (*g*), J. returns to his desire to be big. He would like at least to be medium sized. Note the plastic method of expression used by J. to state this wish. (*h*) How does J. reach this theme ? There is no trace of any associative link. The new theme seems completely spontaneous. J's deliberations about the uncle's nickname are very amusing, it must be admitted. J. is not satisfied with setting up goat and human beings as contrast, but he portrays visually the essentials of the goat.

38

18.2.26. Evening in bed.

T. : " Mama, let us pray softly, so that Baby doesn't wake." (They pray quietly.) " How does the calf drink from the cow ? " (*a*).

M. : " Like this." (She puts T's hand to her mouth.)

T. : " Doesn't it hurt the cow ? " (*b*).

M. : " No."

T. : " Where does the cow get the milk from ? " (c).

M. : " When a cow has a baby, a calf, then she gets milk too, and so do human beings.

T. : " And when all the milk is drunk ? " (d).

M. : " Then some more comes, because the cow drinks."

T. : " Mama, what is bigger than an elephant, but it is not an animal and not a human being ? " (e).

M. : " A church spire."

T. : " Yes."

Discussion.—(a) It is not clear what inner connection could have led T. from praying to this question. It is a case of a spontaneous complex. T. has had ample opportunity to observe how the cow suckles her calf, so his question is not so general as might be expected. Probably the true interpretation of the question is, how does the calf get its nourishment from this process ? That he has a correct idea of the external process is shown indirectly by question (b) ; the idea that suckling a calf might cause the cow pain is a fairly obvious one. Children regard the process as similar to eating or chewing ; that applies at least to the childhood memories of the adults we have questioned on this subject. (c) A question quite natural in the context, and M. utilizes the opportunity to point out in a perfectly natural way the similarity in this respect between man and animals. (d) It is very natural to assume that the cow's milk must get drunk up, just as is the amount of household milk brought daily by the milkman. But the study of milk-production in nature is not pursued, and the conversation takes a quite new turn, by T. asking M. a riddle (e). In the books which were read aloud to the children there were some simple riddles, the solving of which gave great pleasure to the children. This literary model was soon imitated, and often plagiarized a little, but at times quite independent riddles, even if not very elegant ones, were produced. Although it is by no means simple for outsiders to solve these riddles, because of their ambiguity, yet their parents, well acquainted with the structure of the children's thinking, were usually successful. At times the children admitted the correctness of a solution when they had obviously not themselves thought of that solution. In the present case a house for instance would have been a correct solution to the riddle T. asks, but M. suspects that T. means the church-spire, which is the elephant of houses, and pleases him by giving the desired answer.

39

3.3.26. Evening in bed.

T. : " Mama, ask me very softly like a secret if I have done anything." (a).

M. : " Have you done anything to-day ? "

T. : " I cut the towel with the scissors." (b).

M. : " Oh dear, the good new towel ! "

T. : " Only a tiny bit. Did we only get it given to us ? " (c).

M. : " We bought it."

T. : " Can't you buy another one quickly ? " (d).

M. : " No, not so quickly as all that."

Discussion.—(a) The form of the request to be catechized, reveals that T. thinks he has done something very serious, about which he must not speak aloud. But he cannot keep the secret to himself, he must pass it on, for it troubles him greatly. (b) Very early, or as soon as they could use them, we gave the children scissors to cut paper with.[1] They had blunt ends and the children could not harm themselves with them. There is of course always the danger that a valuable article will fall a victim to the scissors, but as experience showed this danger is by no means as great as one would be inclined to suppose. Now such a case had arisen, but on examination, the damage turned out to be much less serious than T. obviously feared. In the interests of the instructive effect the occurrence had to be taken

---

[1] Cf. for this the remarks in Katz, *Erziehung*, p. 60 ff.

as more serious than it really was. Of course it would have been particularly serious if the towel had not belonged to us, but had only been lent, (c) which is what T. probably means by " only given ". (d) The timid question gets a negative reply in order to produce a more lasting effect.

40

5.3.26. Morning in bed.
M. : " Papa has gone away, are you sad ? "
J. : " No."
M. : " Why are you not sad ? "
J. : " Perhaps Papa will write to us that he has packed his things into the bed and done such silly things." (M. had to laugh heartily at this, and J. became thoroughly confused.)

Discussion.—F. had once given the children a comic description of a journey. The books had been packed into bed and he himself had lain on the table, etc. The memory of this comic account prevents J. feeling any grief now at his father's absence.

41

7.3.26. Evening in bed.
J. : " Hans says he won't fight. We may fight with strange children, may we not ? " (a).
M. : " Why do you think Hans won't fight ? "
J. : " He thinks his mother knows (here we have to add to complete the sense ; and doesn't want him to, and so Hans won't) but she doesn't know, and it isn't so serious, is it ? " (b). " It's serious if he falls into the water, then he must write a letter to his mother, but he can't do that, he writes scribble-scrabble, scribble-scrabble you know, up down, up, dot your i, and he can't write noughts either." (c).

Discussion.—Hans is a friend of the children, in age between T. and J. He came for some time every day with his sister Hertha to play with our children. (a) J. is cross that Hans will not fight with him. The reason J. gives for Hans' refusal is quite reasonable ; he thinks Hans won't fight because his mother doesn't allow him to do so (b). J. passes from what is not serious to what appears serious to him (c), e.g. if Hans falls into the water. Now comes an idea of priceless naïveté : Hans must write a letter to his mother. He means this quite seriously ; it is not intended humorously, as the adult feels it. So Hans is to write a letter, but—he can't. Speaking of writing causes J. to be drawn from his original theme by associative connections with this theme. He returns to his starting point only with his last words : Hans also can't write noughts.

42

7.3.26. Evening in bed.

J. : " Mama, you know Auntie O. doesn't clear away at night the things we've been playing with." (a).

M. : " You're telling tales."

J. : " Yes, but Auntie O. must clear away the things." (b).

M. : " No, you yourself must clear them away and not Auntie O."

J. : " Mama, telling tales and lies is nothing." (c).

M. : " One mustn't tell tales and lies."

J. : " But Mama, when Lynx (the landlord's dog) is standing near Zeecks (a shop in the town) and we stand in the garden and call Lynx, then it is a tree and not Lynx." (d).

M. : " Yes, Lynx can't hear you but you know you mustn't tell lies and tales."

J. : " No, we mustn't do that. Mama, now go to Theodor." (e).

M. : " Do you want to go to sleep now ? "

J. : " Yes."

Discussion.—(a, b) We considered it important for the children in the evening before going to bed themselves, to clear away the things they had been playing with. Unfortunately the nursery maids, much against our will, often did this clearing away themselves in order to get finished sooner, so that the children began to think that they had nothing to do with clearing away, which was the nursemaid's job. (c) This statement to which J. proceeds suddenly means probably " telling lies and tales should not be done ", but there is a further meaning " I will have nothing to do with such things ".   When M. has emphasized that one must not tell tales and lies, J. tries in statement (*d*) to construct a case where there is not a lie, but a mistake or delusion. He wants to say " if one is a victim of a delusion, that is not reprehensible ".   The sentence means : if one mistakes a tree for Lynx that is not a lie but a delusion.   J. does not succeed in formulating this, but chooses a much more extensive image, the sense of which must be guessed. (*e*) M. is sent away by J. so that she may have time to talk to T.

43

8.3.26.   Whilst putting on shoes to go out.
J. :   " I want school to last longer." (*a*).
M. :   " Should school last all day ? "
J. :   " Yes."
Hans :   " I want to stay and sleep here too ; I'll sleep with Theodor and Hertha with Baby." (*b*).
Hertha :   " And Auntie O. must undress Hertha." (*c*).
T. :   " And then you'll stay with us all day and all night and drink milk with us." (*d*).
M. :   " If your mother is tired sometime you can stay with us and your mother can rest."
Hans :   " Our mother never gets enough rest." (*e*).

Discussion.—(*a*) The regular daily visits of Hans and Hertha lasted some time and were called " school " by the children.   The four children got on very well together. T. and Hans, J. and Hertha felt happy in this ordered existence and we did not like to separate them.   Thus the desire for school to last longer.   (*b, c*) Hans and Hertha are in favour of a complete removal and T. agrees (*d*). Hans has correctly observed (*e*) that his mother is kept so fully occupied with the children about this time that she never gets enough rest.

44

9.3.26. Forenoon in the nursery.

Hans : (pointing to a wardrobe). " This is the hedge. Theodor, climb on the wardrobe." (a).

T. : " What shall I do ? Shall I climb on the wardrobe ? "

Hans : " Yes."

T. : " Will you help me ? "

Hans : " Yes. Baby, jump from the table." (J. climbs from the table. T. has abandoned the attempt to climb on the wardrobe and has pulled a drawer from the table. He commands all to get in, calling out that they are to take their places in the drawer. Soon they are all sitting in the drawer.)

Hans : " Where are we going ? "

T. : " To Africa."

Hans : " Come, Professor." (b).

Discussion.—We give here a sample of nursery conversations, overheard when the children were talking among themselves. Like other conversations of this kind, it reveals that on these occasions the conversation is much more determined by the situation than when adults take part, and develops chiefly as the situation changes. The child needs the participation of adults in his conversation, to be able to keep to the theme. The conversations of children among themselves are much shorter. Piaget has recorded numerous conversations of children among themselves. He has clearly demonstrated a type of conversation carried on by children in the presence of other children, where the children do indeed make verbal utterances, but do not direct them as replies to the others present. They may be labelled monologues in which several persons participate. But we are not dealing with this type of conversation in the present case. The children *do* intend to affect each other by their conversation, they *are* talking to each other and are trying mutually to bring each other to perform some action. The logical connection between the verbal utterances is here made through the medium of the game they are playing together, the individual stages of which they discuss among themselves. There is no need to enter into any lengthy discussion—we will only mention two points. (*a*) In the game the wardrobe represents to Hans a hedge, but he calls it quite correctly a wardrobe when he orders T. to climb on it, for if he said hedge it would not be understood. (*b*) They are Professor's children and so the title—*wie die Alten sungen*.

45

9.3.26.   Evening in bed.
J. : " Mama, I always dream something nasty and then I try to think of something nice. Mama, why can't I dream about what I try to ? " (*a*).
M. : " Why, what do you dream about ? "
J. : " I don't know. I've forgotten." (*b*).
T. : " I dream nasty things too." (*c*).
J. : " Mama, I dreamt that an elephant has two legs, isn't that funny ? Of course an elephant has four legs." (*d*).
T. : " But a stork has two legs like a human being." (*e*). (In the meantime J. has fallen asleep.)
M. : " And what do you dream about ? "
T. : " I don't know. I've forgotten." (*f*).

Discussion.—(*a*) It does not seem very probable to us that J. has really made an effort to influence his " nasty " dreams by trying to think of something nice. Perhaps J. has heard at some time of the possibility of such influence, and now he speaks about it as though he had really tried it. We could not discover with certainty whether any one had spoken to him about such a possibility, but we are quite sure there had been no mention of it by us. (*b*) First of all J. declares he cannot remember any dream, but then (*c*) he goes on to report one. We cannot say for certain whether it is really a dream or only imagination helped by the frequent picture book illustrations of elephants walking on their hind legs. Whatever the case, an elephant with two legs is a very possible childish dream motive. (*c*) It is very probable that T's statement about the nastiness of his dreams is quite true. At this time we often had the impression that

T. was disturbed by his dreams. (*e*) At this moment the similarity between men and storks as two-legged creatures occurs to T. (*f*) Even an adult when asked suddenly is usually unable to mention a previous dream.

46

10.3.26. Evening in bed. Negroes had been discussed.
T. : " Negroes have a black skin, but their teeth are white. Mama, you know their teeth look so specially white only because their skin is so black. Negroes teeth are just as white as our teeth I think."

Discussion.—Although this is rather a monologue than a conversation, we include it because of its convincing proof of the appearance of contrast and because of its explanation. We must stress that T. came quite independently to his conclusion and to the theoretical statement following. Neither by us, nor, certainly, by anyone else had his attention been drawn to contrast phenomena in general or to the special case at issue here.[1]

47

13.3.26. Morning.
M. : " Auntie O., the children must come to breakfast. It is already ten o'clock."
O. : " My watch says only half past nine."
M. : " My husband's watch says ten, as well as mine. I think that's right."
T. : " Yes Mama, Auntie O's watch is wrong."
M. : " Why do you think so ? "
T. : " Well because two watches say ten o'clock and only one says half past nine."

Discussion.—Here we have a correct conclusion arrived at inductively. If two watches show the same time, then it is more probable that *they* show the correct time than that

[1] According to other evidence children are quite likely to notice contrast appearances very early. Cf. D. Katz, *Studien zur Kinderpsychologie*, Leipzig, 1913 ; G. Révész, " Ueber spontane und systematische Selbstbeobachtung bei Kindern," *Zeitschr. angew. Psychol.*, vol. 21, 1923.

one watch showing a different time does so. The spontaneous conclusion, formulated when asked for, reveals a good thinking capacity.

48

15.3.26. Afternoon.
M. : " Where have you been this afternoon ? "
T. : " In Barnstorf."
M. : " And we walked to Gehlsdorf and came back on the ferry."
J. : " Did you walk as far as Denmark ? " (a).
M. : " No, not as far as Denmark, that would have been rather far."
T. : " It would have been too far." (b).

Discussion.—The children know that the ferry from Warnemünde goes to Denmark, and have already been in Denmark with their parents. (a) It only needs mention of the ferry to convince J. that we had been to Denmark on it. J. has already been to Gehlsdorf on the small ferry-boats, but that had not made the same impression on him as the big ferry to Denmark. M's joking remark that Denmark would be rather far is made more precise by T's conclusion that it would have been too far. (b).

49

18.3.26. Evening in bed.
J. : " Mama, Hans says ' mittenkins '. There isn't such a thing, is there ? " (a).
M. : " Yes there is."
J. : " In the shop near the Steintor there are some balloons and Hans says ' mittenkins '. That's not right, is it ? " (b).
M. : " Oh, balloons are to fly and mittens are to warm the hands."
J. : " To warm soldiers, but there are balloons near the Steintor." (c).
M. : " Let us pray now."
J. : " Yes."
T. : " I want to pray too, to pray badly." (d).

M. : " We must pray well." (They pray.) " Good-night, Julius."

T. : " Mama, now come to me."

J. : " Mama, go to Theodor now or else he'll fall asleep."

Discussion.—(*a, b, c*) Hans' word " mittenkins " has had a strong effect on J. He must already have heard of mittens, or he would not know that soldiers wear them for warmth ; it must be the diminutive form of the word which intrigues him. This form seems so strange to him that he disputes the very existence of the word itself and of the thing designated by the word, for the two are not sharply distinguished by children. But there is something else. Probably on the usual daily walk Hans with his customary habit of playing with a word has called all kinds of things " mittenkins ", the balloons included. This has distressed J. and he is now striving to help the balloons to their right to a special name. (*d*) Because M. usually says " let us pray well " T. is driven in his exuberance to say he will pray badly. It is very rare that T. reveals such negativism as he does here, and it is not to be taken seriously.

50

20.3.26. Forenoon.

M. : " Did you look for Theodor yesterday when he was in Warnemünde ? "

J. : " When I'm big I'll take a key and walk to Warnemünde and not take you with me because you didn't take me." (*a*).

M. : " You are still too small."

J. : " That doesn't matter (*b*). (J. is almost weeping and pulls such a comic face that M. cannot repress a slight smile. This offends J. and he attempts to strike M.)

M. : " You mustn't strike. Boys don't strike."

J. : " I'll go to America and pull my boat ashore and then you can't come on it." (*c*).

T. : " But we'll come after you." (*d*).

M. : (to disarm J. by kindness). " We'll go on ahead and when you reach America we'll be already there and we'll wave our handkerchiefs to you."

I

J. : " Then I'll tie a motor-boat to my boat and other boats too." (e).

T. : " Then the people will make fun of you." (f).

M. : (to change the subject). " Only Vikings did that."

T. : " Mama, who were they ? "

M. : " You know in Denmark and other countries the king's eldest son always got the kingdom and the other sons sailed away in their ships and became pirates. When they saw a ship they used to jump overboard and take the finest things for themselves."

T. : " Mama, what does ' overboard ' mean ? " (g).

M. : " Your bed has a board at the bottom and ships have an end like your bed, this end is called ' board ' on ships. Can you remember, you've seen a board on ships ? "

T. : " Yes—Mama, are there pirates still ? " (h).

M. : " No, people decided that no one should attack another person."

T. : " Did the pirates try again ? " (j).

M. : " Yes at first they tried again, but they were punished and didn't do it again."

T. : " Have Auntie and Uncle R. (in Copenhagen) seen pirates too ? " (k).

M. : " No."

Discussion.—The parents had been to Warnemünde with T., but as J. was still sleeping when the start was made, he was left at home. J. feels hurt by this and now describes how he will take his revenge for the slight he has suffered. (a) He will take a key, to him the symbol of being grown up. His desire to be someone (b) is offended by the statement that he is too small, and he tries to prove his strength by a blow. Then he continues with his imaginary revenge (c, e) and develops a truly childish boastful display of strength. He thinks the more boats and motor-boats he takes on his expedition, the greater the impression he will make. T. rouses him still further by his remark (d), and is fully appreciative of the comic side of the America expedition (f). M. now gives a fresh orientation to the conversation which by this time is distressing J. She mentions the Vikings, knowing very well that both children will be attracted, and at once all ill-feeling vanishes. (g) A good question, which seizes the unfamiliar term " overboard " and asks its meaning. (h, j) These questions are not due to anxiety, but on the contrary pirates have the fullest sympathy of both children. (k) Why does T. connect pirates with Auntie and Uncle R. in Copenhagen ? The journey to Copenhagen had meant the children's first long sea-voyage, so that T. fixes the pirates' home on the sea he knows, and thereby indirectly they are connected with the Danish acquaintances.

51

21.3.26. Evening in bed.

T. : " Mama, did the Vikings jump overboard on the ferry ? " (a).

M. : " Perhaps they did if they thought they could get something."

T. : " Or perhaps someone had told them they ought to jump back again and they were seeing if they could do it." (b).

M. : " It is possible, Theodor. I can't really say. In any case we can now journey wherever we want and need have no fear of being attacked by pirates."

T. : " Or else one might travel by railway." (c).

M. : " There wasn't any railway then. Do you know who invented it ? "

T. : " No."

M. : " It was Stephenson. When he was a little boy he was sitting with his mama and he saw how the kettle-lid was lifted when the water inside the kettle began to boil, and so he thought steam could move things. Then he got an engine worked by steam and made it draw a train."

T. : " Did he build a little train first ? " (d).

M. : " Yes. People made fun of him at first and said steam couldn't move anything, but then they saw it could."

T. : " First of all they'd built trains for men and then later on cattle-trucks and milk-vans." (e).

M. : " Yes. Before there were any railways, people used to use horses, donkeys, camels, and elephants."

T. : " And they went to America by ship and when there was ice they used to walk." (f).

M. : " But you know the sea does not freeze everywhere. Where it's warm it doesn't freeze at all."

T. : " Mama, and the little wagons which carry sand on rails (tipping wagons), did Stephenson invent those ? " (g).

M. : " No, gradually everybody found out something."

T. : " Did Papa find out anything ? " (h).

M. : " Yes, Papa discovered the vibratory sense."

T. : " Vibratory sense ? " (j).

M. : " Yes, when a heavy cart goes past the house then the ground trembles under our feet ; we call that vibrating."

T. : " Does everybody know that now ? " (k).

M. : " Many people do."

T. : " Did people at first make fun of him ? " (l)

M. : " No, people don't make fun of others so quickly now.   We see with our eyes, that is called the sense of sight. What do we hear with ? "

T. and J. : " With our ears."

M. : " That is called the sense of hearing.   What do we smell with ? "

T. and J. : " With our noses."

M. : " That is called the sense of smell.   And what do we taste with ? "

T. and J. : " With our mouths."

M. : " With our tongue, and we call that the sense of taste.   And the sense with which we notice vibration when a heavy cart goes past is called the vibratory sense."

T. : " Did Papa notice that poor people's houses shake when carts go past ? " (m).

M. : " No, Theodor, you can notice that in every house."

Discussion.—(a) Once the Vikings have aroused the children's imagination they continue to play a very important part.   Having decided that the sphere of their activities was the Danish waters (conv. 50), T. naturally concludes that they also must have paid a visit at some time to the big railway ferry.   The dangerous element in the pirates was not understood, and T. tends to look on their activities more from the point of view of sport (b) and thinks it must be an amusing game to jump overboard and then to jump back again. (c) The idea that one might travel by railway to avoid the pirates shows good reasoning power ; T. of course cannot know that there were no railways at the time of the Vikings. The conversation takes a new turn through M's remark about the invention of the steam-engine. For some time now T. had shown a great interest in technical things, an interest which is probably always present in boys of this age. Whenever he found an opportunity he used to watch machines working, and was extremely reluctant to leave them. The elementary explanation of the principle of the action of steam was exactly suited to his interests and capacity. (d) From the child's standpoint it is extremely probable that Stephenson first built a small train as a toy. (e) That passenger coaches should precede cattle trucks, and these in their turn be made before milk vans, reveals the degree of importance attached by T. to these three categories of vehicle, and may indeed correspond to actual historical fact. (f) T. has heard that the Baltic sometimes freezes over such a large area that one can walk over it. This fact is now made to apply also to the voyage to America. (g) With this question T. returns to Stephenson. T. had been greatly interested in sand-loading at Warnemünde by means of tipping waggons. Perhaps, he thinks, these too, which really are connected with railways, were also invented by Stephenson. (h) Papa, at the moment T's determining ideal, must also have invented something. (The subsequent fragment of conversation, more in the nature of a test, was really recorded for our own personal use. Our excuse for publishing it is that it was the cause of T. producing several charming expressions about the vibratory sense, both here and later in the last conversation recorded.) (k, l) It would have been very painful to T. if his father had been ridiculed. The ensuing lecture in sense psychology is heard by the children with great attention and obvious pleasure. (m) A thoroughly sound process of thought, that vibration (shaking) could be best observed in poor people's houses, which are not so well constructed.

52

31.3.26. The children had just received new drinking cups. F. had told them that the cups, filled with sweets, had been placed outside the door by the Easter Hare. The following conversation ensued.

T. : " Mama, what was the Easter Hare like ? Was he black ? We didn't meet him on the way. He must be a living hare, not a stuffed one, for a stuffed hare can't carry them. Perhaps he'll come back for the cups and fill them up again to-morrow." (a).

M. : " Oh, the Easter Hare would have too much to do if he came to the same family every day."

J. : " Just look, there are some caramel bonbons in the cup."

T. : (correcting him) " Cream bonbons."

J. : " Cream bonbons."

T. : " Mama, it smells of soap." (b). (Under the eggs was some shavings on which soap had been lying.)

G. : " Perhaps the Hare had it near some soap he was taking to someone else."

T. : " Mama, I know now, you wrote on the invitation (some children had been invited to a party) that the Easter Hare had promised to be present, and that's why he came (c). At R's (a friend's) there is a big Easter Hare, but I think it's made of wood."

M. : " You've also got a new toothbrush."

T. : " From the Easter Hare too ? " (d).

M. : " Or perhaps from Wertheim's ? "

T. : " Or Wertheim's put it into the Easter Hare's basket and he brought it here." (e).

J. : " The Easter Hare is my friend because he was here. I've known him for quite a long time." (f).

G. : " Perhaps the Easter Hare is sitting in Wertheim's, where the bear was before."

J. : " I've known the Easter Hare ever since Copenhagen. Perhaps the Easter Hare will bring me a whole shop." (g).

Discussion.—We found the poetry of the Easter Hare so entertaining to the children that we had no scruples in introducing him as the bringer of presents at Easter time, and in crediting him with being the layer of eggs. This temporary distortion of natural facts can scarcely do any great damage, such as we know, for instance, results from the Stork fairy tale. The Easter Hare can be spoken about in such a way that the children feel the diversion from natural fact to be merely a humorous addition. Everything connected with the Easter Hare filled the children with such joy that we considered it compatible with our pedagogical conscience to let the Easter Hare become a reality, even at the risk of temporary scientific confusion. We have never seen the children so full of unalloyed happiness as they were in the following situation. F. borrowed from a colleague a charming little rabbit, very similar to a hare in colour. A nest of green paper strips was made on a cover in the hall at home, and the rabbit was placed in this, surrounded by a number of gaily coloured eggs of different sizes. The rabbit did us the honour of remaining perfectly still in its nest. We then told the children that the Easter Hare had come to see them, and they were to come down to the hall and look. When the children saw the live Easter Hare sitting amongst the eggs they were literally speechless with amazement and joy. All who witnessed this boundless happiness were quite sure that no adult is ever capable of such unalloyed bliss. The live Easter Hare remained our guest for some days and the children built a house for him and looked after him most carefully. At a children's party which we gave shortly afterwards, the live Easter Hare was the sole centre of attraction. It was a charming spectacle ; the hare on the table and all the children grouped around him. Of course we had to take care that the children's frequent manifestations of love did not harm the animal. The foregoing conversation took place some days before the meeting with the live Easter Hare just described. (a) With regard to the Easter Hare, T. is hovering between belief and doubt, until the impression made by the presents causes him for the moment to be more inclined to believe. How splendid it would be if the hare were to call for the cups and bring them back, once they had been emptied ! (b) Another proof of T's excellent nose. The eggs had as a matter of fact a slight smell of the soap which had been wrapped in the shavings. (c) T. now remembers the invitation to the party sent to some of his friends. Now it is clear why the Easter Hare came. (d, e) What a mixture of imagination and reality. M. brings the well-known Wertheim's store into the conversation in order to test T., but once his imagination is set on fire, the store becomes woven into the Easter Hare's activities. (f, g) Since even the elder brother is now convinced, it is no wonder that J. is absolutely enchanted by the Easter Hare. Best of all he would like to make the Easter Hare his brother, because he brought such lovely presents. Then it occurs to him that he saw a real hare in a garden in Copenhagen and this one is now identified with the Easter Hare. Especially in J's case we have had ample opportunity to observe an inclination, under the stimulus of pleasure, to mingle together what he knows and what he desires.

53

6.4.26. Morning at breakfast.

T. : " Was God born ? " (a).

M. : " I'll tell you when you are bigger."

T. : " God created all men, didn't he, so he must have been born himself." (b).

M. : " God wasn't born and God doesn't die, he can't be seen and heard ; I'll tell you how when you are bigger."

T. : " If God doesn't die, then all men won't die." (c).

M : " I'll tell you all about that when you are bigger."

T. : " You shouldn't say things like that, it's rude." (d).

F. : (fondles him) " You little metaphysician."

T. : (considers awhile, obviously seeking a term of abuse with which he can reply to metaphysician) " You crocodile ! " (e).

Discussion.—An important theological conversation ! (a) This question confirms what we have previously stated about the child's tendency to make the idea of God concrete (conv. 32). (b) Without letting M. divert him from his theme, T. continues with his rational consideration on theology. It is his burning interest in the subject which causes him to persist so obstinately. (c) This statement, so to speak the reverse of (b), is contained either explicitly or implicitly in every system of rational theology. The fact that a child only five years old is able to formulate it without any external stimulus, but merely from his own speculation, causes one to think very hard. (d) It displeases T. not to receive immediately a clear answer to questions which occupy him so completely. He does not want to be put off by promises, and so his father's friendly " metaphysician " meant as praise is answered by abuse. The child does not understand " metaphysician ", and we may have quite valid grounds for doubting whether his epithet is equivalent to the term used by his father.

54

6.4.26. Afternoon. In the train from Warnemünde to Rostock.

F. : (asks in fun) " Has the railway-coach any eyes ? "
T. : " Yes, the buffers." (a).
F. : " And its mouth ? "
T. : " That is the line underneath (b)." (He means the horizontal line below the buffers).
F. : (pointing to the luggage-rack). " And that ? "
T. : " Is the brain." (c).
F. : " The arms ? "
T. : " The doors." (d).
F. : " The legs ? "
T. : " The wheels." (e).
F. : " The father ? "
T. : " The engine." (f).
F. : " The mother ? "
T. : " The tender." (g).
F. : " What does the train eat ? "
T. : " People, which he spits out again." (h). (After considering some time.) " The other trains are his brothers." (j).

Discussion.—This must be termed a test conversation in

the sense previously stated. (*a*) After T. had at once given a most appropriate answer to the first joking question (by the way, F. had expected as answer " the lights " but the buffers, especially as there are two of them, do look like eyes) F. carried on the humorous questioning, in order to test T's capacity to make analogies. Question and answer succeeded each other rapidly. T. took a real pleasure in this intellectual game, so similar to riddle guessing, and his eyes began to sparkle. (*b*) The conversation took place in the train, and so the answer was given without T. seeing the coach and the buffers before him. He must previously have noted the similarity to a face without having expressed it in words. (*c*) The reference to the luggage-rack was made hurriedly, without really expecting T. to find an analogy. If an adult had given the same reply as T., it would have been natural to suppose an analogy between the network of the rack and of the nervous system. T's *tertium comparationis* is probably the " above " of the rack and of the brain. (*d, e*) The comparisons arms-doors and legs-wheels are good, the former being a particularly worthy performance. (*f*) Father —engine must be accounted a skilful achievement, and (*g*) Mother—tender is also an apt analogy, but (*h*) is even better. This answer came quite unexpectedly, for the reply " coal " was much more obvious. T. has certainly never heard of such a comparison ; we have a quite new creative performance. The spontaneous final remark (*j*) may be classed as quite appropriate.[1]

55

14.4.26. After a meal, when T. was to rest in bed.

M. : " *Robinson Crusoe* is a fine book, let me read it to you."

[1] *Re* the whole of this conversation, cf. Werner's remarks about the importance of physiognomy in the child's mental life. In all cases he says, the physiognomy is the original factor, and the specific-human element is only a special case. The child's world of perception is a world of physiognomy. (Werner, p. 53 and p. 104.)

T. : " Before, I used to say Berni (by Scharrelmann) is the finest book, but now I say *Robinson Crusoe* is the finest book. Later on I'll say another book is the finest."

M. : " No, you know *Robinson Crusoe* is always a fine book. Many people say children need no other books but *Robinson Crusoe.*"

Discussion.—One must have experienced what *Robinson Crusoe* can mean to a child in order to understand Rousseau's demand that *Robinson Crusoe* should be the only book given to children to read. T. was enchanted by readings from this classic, not once, but time and again. He lived wholly with Crusoe, and shared all his adventures, all his joys and sorrows. In the first statement M. is referring to T's frequently expressed opinion that *Robinson Crusoe* is the finest book. T's answer reveals a self criticism which does him all honour, a self criticism not met with in all adults.[1] How often one meets people who, continually talking in superlatives, always regard the last book they have read as the best, and their latest amusement as the most enjoyable. It is true that T. had been fascinated by the contents of Scharrelmann's Berni, and had been convinced that Berni was really a living boy. The illustrations in the book helped towards this illusion as they were expressly intended for children. T. shared all Berni's adventures. We cannot say whether T. had actually spoken of Berni as the finest book he had yet met, but probably he felt it to be so, even without formulating his opinion in words. And now when he comes to confess that Crusoe is the finest book, he discovers that these two opinions cannot be reconciled. And not only that, he is dissatisfied with himself for having to change his mind so quickly. He fears that another change of opinion will take place later on, and has no confidence that he will not then claim a third book as the finest. It was quite in order here for M. to make the

---

[1] E. Köhler (p. 58) gives an example of self criticism at a still earlier age. Ännchen (2 years, 6 months) says : " I cannot speak it, I'm so dull ! "

consoling statement that many people consider Crusoe as the most valuable of all books for children.

56

17.4.26.   Evening in bed.

J. : " When I go to the Gomnasium (Gymnasium) I will make good progress and people will think I am Wilhelm (a friend who had gone to the Gymnasium at Easter) (*a*). And then they'll ask : ' Are you Wilhelm ? ' And I'll say : ' I'm Theodor.' " (*b*).

M. : " But are you Theodor ? "

J. : " They'll ask me, then I'll say I'm Fritz Gras (a name of J's own invention"). (*c*).

M. : " Why don't you want to say that you are Julius Gregor ? "

J. : " When I am big, I won't be Julius any more ; the children will say : ' Julius Pulius,' then I won't be Julius Gregor any more, I'll be Theodor then." (*d*).

Discussion.—The fundamental motive of J's utterances in this conversation is once again his desire to be of some importance, a desire which is stronger in him, the younger child, than in his elder brother. Although we tried our utmost to treat both children exactly alike and not to favour either, so as not to arouse any feeling of inferiority in J., yet the mere difference in age caused distinct differences in performance which J. noticed and which caused his manly protest. T. could do many things impossible to J., merely because of his superior size : he could reach higher objects and climb on to higher articles of furniture. He could perform many manual operations beyond J's capacity with his less developed dexterity. T. could understand many conversations carried on in the children's presence, whereas J's powers of understanding did not yet go so far. These natural circumstances could not be avoided, and hence arose the source of J's grief, the fact that he was not equal in capacity to his brother. F. was T's ideal, but J's dearest wish was to be like T. In the present conversation at first (*a*) J. expresses his desire to go like his friend Wilhelm to the Gymnasium, around which a certain halo hovers. Surreptitiously associative tendencies turn the friend Wilhelm into the brother Wilhelm, for only from the latter does the way lead to the second name Theodor, which he will give to people when asked (*b*). But this turn is not enough for the rogue. Theodor becomes Fritz Gras, (*c*) a person invented by J. on the spur of the moment, for the surname Gras does not occur amongst any of our acquaintances. Most surprising of all is the last statement (*d*). J. is convinced that when he is big he will no longer be Julius and be called Julius Gregor, but he will be Theodor. He *would like* to be Theodor and he *will* be Theodor. The law of the inviolability of the identity of personalities troubles him just as little as it does the Red Indian who is at one and the same time a parrot. In the last remark we have an interlude produced by the play of sounds Julius-Pulius.[1] As far as we know the word Pulius had never been used before. It represents a humorous momentary improvisation which J. could not resist.

We would point out that J's utterances in this conversation are determined largely by association. If they were but a little less ordered we should have a " salad of words ". We see quite clearly how purely associative tendencies break through the structure of logically connected series of thoughts.

57

18.4.26. Afternoon.

T. : " Papa, if you were a woman would you like to have your hair like Auntie M. ? " (*a*).

F. : " Isn't Mama's hair nicer ? "

T. : " Yes, well in between (*b*). Papa, the Chinese have beautiful eyes, placed like this (makes a gesture to show slanting). Papa, if you had eyes like a Chinese your spectacles would have to be like them too (i.e. slanting)." (*c*).

Discussion.—(*a*) Auntie M. had visited us some days previously. She was the first lady with bobbed hair that

---

[1] Cf. " Georgie-Porgie " (English nursery rhyme).

T. had been able to scrutinize closely. So his question really is, whether F. would like to have bobbed hair, if he were a woman. It is not easy to see what caused T. to address such a question to his father ; it would have been more reasonable to suppose that he would ask his mother, who was not following the new fashion. T. is confused by F's reference to M's hair. He thinks (*b*) that one should have a style of hairdressing midway between his mother's (for whatever M. has or does is right and good) and that of Auntie M. which has also impressed him. So T. arrives at the strange way out of his confusion determined by moral and æsthetic means. (*c*) " Beautiful " has probably no æsthetic meaning in this context, but is only used to characterize the pecularity of expression known to T. from pictures. The proposal about the spectacles is in itself sensible, for slanting eyes do need slanting spectacles to look through.

58

19.4.26.   Afternoon.

T. : (discovers a tooth-pick on F's desk) " Oh, I'd like that."

F. : " What do you want it for ? "

T. : " What do you do with it ? "

F. : (joking) " I pin up my troubles with it."

T. : (laughing) " I want to pin my troubles up with it too." (*a*).

F. : " Why have you any troubles ? What troubles have you ? "

T. : " I shan't tell you." (*b*).

F. : " Well, what are troubles ? "

T. : " Troubles are thoughts." (*c*).

F. : " Have you ever seen them ? "

T. : " They can't be seen." (*d*).

Discussion.—(*a*) T. understands the humour of his father's remark, and falls in with the mood. (*b, c*) T. can scarcely know what troubles are from his own experience, but their grandmother had often told the children about her sad experiences and probably added that those were her troubles.

Troubles and thoughts seem to be synonymous to T., but he will not reveal his thoughts. (*d*) This last remark is very good. Thoughts cannot be seen, i.e. perceived by the senses, that is their particular quality.

59

30.4.26. Evening in bed.

T. : " I'd much rather go to Miss D. (i.e. to a preparatory school run by Miss D., and not to the elementary school). You only need stay three years there." (*a*).

M. : " If possible you'll go to Miss D's, if not to St. George's School. Perhaps you need only stay three years there."

T. : " Is Wilhelm (conv. 56) now at a Realgymnasium ? "

M. : " No, he is at the Gymnasium.[1] There they teach Greek and Latin, but less mathematics and no chemistry at all."

T. : " But I want to learn Greek and Kiki." (*b*).

M. : " Chemistry."

T. : " Yes, chemistry, but Greek as well. I want to learn mathematics as well. I want to go to the Gymnasium and to the Realgymnasium." (*c*).

J. : " It's such a long time since we heard any soldiers' songs." (*d*).

M. : " Papa wanted to sing to you this evening, but we were out."

J. : " You were out for a walk, if people don't go for a walk they die." (*e*).

T. : " People don't die if they don't go for a walk, but they grow pale and if they go for a walk they get rosy cheeks." (*f*).

Discussion.—Recently there had been much talk about T. going to school. He would not be six until November of this year, so of course he could not go at Easter. The parents had discussed both the possibility of attending a private preparatory school and the elementary school. (*a*) It is somewhat surprising that T. has grasped the difference in time of attendance between the two schools, and is already showing a disinclination for the elementary school, where

[1] The German Gymnasium means a Grammar School.

he will have to remain one year longer. (*b*, *c*) T. of course has not the slightest idea of the difference between a classical and a modern education, and has just as little conception of the terms Greek, Chemistry, and Mathematics. His remarks probably mean that he desires to learn as much as possible at school, and to let nothing escape him. Therefore attendance at a Gymnasium and Realgymnasium simultaneously. (*d*) Spontaneously, with no recognizable associative bridge, J. expresses the wish to hear once more the songs which F. sometimes used to sing to the children at night before they went to sleep ; for the most part they were songs of a humorous nature. (*e*) In order to accustom the children to taking walks regularly we had told them that fresh air was essential to health, and this J. exaggerates into the statement that one would die otherwise. T. proceeds to give a somewhat lengthy correction of this statement. (*f*).

60

23.4.26. A friend of ours, a teacher in a boy's school, had permitted T. on occasion to come into the lowest class, which he taught, and to remain during the lesson. These visits gave the greatest pleasure to T. To-day M. has met the child at school and the following conversation develops.

M. : " Could the other children paint better than you ? "

T. : " Other children shall not paint better than I, I want to (be able to) paint best of all." (*a*).

M. : " Theodor, perhaps you can do other things better instead."

T. : " What could I do better ? " (*b*).

M. : " You know *Robinson Crusoe* and all kinds of stories, which other children don't know."

Discussion.—(*a*) For the first time T. here reveals himself clearly to be ambitious. This characteristic had scarcely been suspected by us previously. Obviously to bring out this trait an adequate stimulus was needed, that of the presence of children of equal age to him, who were perhaps superior at the work required. His ambition now appears undisguised in the desire—or rather the demand—that other children shall not paint better than he. By saying he can do many things better than other children M. consoles him in order to avoid any feelings of inferiority (educating up to the "courage to be incomplete" is only in place at a much later age—perhaps). But T. is suspicious, he wants to know what he can do better (b). M's information seems to satisfy him.

61

23.4.26. Afternoon. On the occasion of his first going to school (previous conversation) T. has been given a bag of sweets. On returning from school he had given the bag to F. to keep, and would ask for some of the contents from time to time. The bag lay always, just as on this occasion, on F's writing desk.

F. : "When I look at your bag I always think of you."

T. : "When I go away I think of you too, but when I am in school then I've forgotten you." (a).

F. : (half in fun) "I never forget you and you forget me."

T. : "I must put something that looks like you on the table in school, then I'll think of you. I must place your spectacles on the table, then I shan't forget you." (b).

Discussion.—(a) Noteworthy as an observation of experience. When he has just taken his departure he still thinks of Father, but in school, with its many new impressions he doesn't think of him. T. is honest enough not to conceal his forgetting. (b) T's means of keeping F. in mind is that of a visible sign. The phrase "something that looks like you" is splendid ; it means "something belonging to you which reminds me of you". The spectacles are not only an external reminder of F. but are indeed a part of Father because they "look like him".

62

25.4.26. Afternoon, at table. T. takes F's hand and feels it above and below. Of late T. has often taken F's hand and said lovingly "Papa's hand is warm and rough".[1]

T. : "Papa, I love you 'two'."

[1] "A human being loves as a complete man. . . . And so a child's love is permeated with instincts to touch physically." (Stern, p. 468.)

F. : " What does that mean ? "

T. : " Your hand is warm on top and cold underneath."

F. : " How do you love Mama ? "

T. : " When Mama's hand is warm on top and under-neath I love her ' one '.   When your hand is cold on top and underneath I love you ' three '."

Discussion.—T. had heard of school report marks and now uses them as a measure of his love.   A curious idea. What is the method ?   It depends on the hand of the beloved person.   The warmer the hand, the greater his love.   If the hand is warm above and below ; Division 1, one side cold ; Division 2, both sides cold ; Division 3.

63

27.4.26.   Midday at table.

T. : " Was Uncle Julius in Africa or America ? "

F. : " In Africa."

T. : " Where the negroes are ? "

F. : " Yes."

T. : " Was he black too ? " (*a*).

F. : " No."

T. : " But if he had gone there as a baby, would he have been black then ? " (*b*).

F. : " No.   To be black the parents must be black too. If Mama and Papa went to Africa and had a baby there it would be white too."

T. : " But Uncle Julius was brown in Africa, wasn't he ? " (*c*).

F. : " Yes, a little."

T. : " And that went away again—why are negroes really black then ? " (*d*).

F. : " Because the sun is so hot where they live."

T. : " Did Uncle Julius go about naked ? " (*e*).

F. : " No, only the negroes go about naked in Africa."

Discussion.—The children had a most unusual interest in negroes, and once again they returned in their conversation to the black people.   The interest in Uncle Julius is probably due in part to their interest in negroes, since Uncle Julius had been amongst the negroes.   (*a*) T. has seen Uncle Julius and knows that he is no longer black, but perhaps he was black in Africa, thinks T. Both children about this time believed that if negroes were thoroughly washed or rubbed down with a cloth, the colour would come off, and they could not be brought to give up this idea. So Uncle Julius too may have gradually lost his African colour by washing. (b) A good question. If one only lives long enough in Africa, one will become black. (c) T. cannot be made to change his opinion so easily. If Uncle Julius was not black, then at least he was brown perhaps? And just as T's brown colour caused by the sun on the beach at Warnemünde gradually disappeared, perhaps Uncle Julius slowly became white again. (d) T. once more returns to the question of negroes with a fundamental question. He accepts unchallenged the answer, which is seemingly at variance with other replies given by F. F., however, found it psychologically more easily comprehensible for the child to connect the sun, and not race, with the colour of the negroes. (e) This assumption by the child is very understandable.

64

1.5.26. Evening in bed. The bell rings.
M. : " I must ask who has just rung."
J. : (when M. returns) " Who was it ? "
M. : " A letter for Papa."
J. : " Did the letter ring ? " (a).
M. : " No, the postman rang."
J. : " Are letters delivered in the evening too ? "
M. : " If they are express letters they are delivered in the evening."
J. : " Otherwise in the mornings ? "
M. : " Yes."
J. : " And if they don't come in the mornings ? " (b).
M. : " Then they come at noon."
J. : " And if the postman does not bring them at noon, then he is naughty, then we'll go to him and take all his letters from him." (c).

Discussion.—(a) The question is quite serious; J. has

no intention of joking. So he thinks it possible for the letter to have rung the bell, probably because M. spoke not quite correctly of a letter, and not of the postman in reply to the question " Who was it ". (b, c) In the course of the conversation it appears that J. thinks people have just as definite a claim to a certain quantity of letters as to the morning milk or rolls, and in M's replies there is indeed no mention of only potential letters to be received. So J's anger against the postman increases—he is naughty, all his letters must be taken from him if he will not deliver those to which people have a just claim.

65

6.5.26.   J. has had his afternoon nap and has just wakened.

M. : " Did you dream about anything ? "

J. : " No, I didn't dream at all."

T. : " Didn't you dream that you were hovering ? " (a).

J. : " No."

M. : " Theodor, do you dream that you are hovering ? "

T. : " Yes, with an aeroplane to heaven and there is no angel there, a little baby pig was there, it was a little sucking pig." (b).

Discussion.—It is very probable from the spontaneous and precise way in which T. formulates the question to his brother, that he knows from personal experience the dream of flying, which has caused so much discussion in works on dreams. Such a dream had never been discussed in his presence. The expression " hover " too vouches for the truth of his dream ; this word is very seldom used with reference to the processes of every-day life. We cannot discuss whether the particulars with which T. adorns his account are accurate. The fact that it is almost certain that a five year-old child had this dream of flying, strengthens our suspicions as to the reliability of the interpretation of the " dream of flying " as a sexual-erotic dream and makes a physiological explanation (overcoming sensation of weight) more probable.

66

7.5.26. Early morning in bed.

T. : " What is wool made of ? "

M. : " Wool grows on sheep."

T. : (points to the feather-bed) " And is that filled with wool ? "

M. : " No, the feather-bed is not filled with wool, but with feathers."

T. : " Whenever the man finds a feather he takes it and collects feathers for a bed."

M. : " Yes, feathers are collected for a feather-bed."

T. : " But a great many must be collected, for feathers are only found in ones." (*a*).

M. : " The feathers are taken from dead birds."

T. : " Yes, then one has a whole pile at once. And have the Eskimos feather-beds too ? " (*b*).

M. : " No, they use skins as coverings."

T. : " And what are their cushions made of ? "

M. : " They place skins under their heads."

T. : " And they make their clothes of skins, I know that." (*c*).

F. : " And do you know where Eskimos carry their children ? "

T. : " Where ? "

M. : " On their backs in rucksacks. Just imagine if Papa were to carry you, and I Julius, and your heads peeped out."

T. : " The Eskimos have their kitchens on their sleighs or on the ship, like in Warnemünde ; there are ships there with kitchens." (*d*).

M. : " Yes, in Warnemünde there are ships with kitchens, but the Eskimos make a fire when they stop, they don't have kitchens on their sleighs."

T. : " Are the Eskimos a different colour from us ? "

F. : " Why do you think so ? "

T. : " Negroes are black and it's so cold where the Eskimos live—are the Eskimos blue ? " (*e*).

F. : " No, the Eskimos are similar in colour to us, perhaps a little browner."

T. : " What are the Eskimos' houses like ? "

F. : " Their houses are made of snow."

T. : " And what do the Eskimos make their spades of ? "

M. : " The Eskimos aren't like Robinson Crusoe, they can travel farther and exchange their skins for spades."

Discussion.—(*a*) The children had collected feathers on their walks, and so T. thinks it must be very laborious to get together the feathers for a feather-bed. (*b*) Robinson Crusoe was T's daily reading-matter about this time. The same thing which so attracted T. in Crusoe, that is the primitive way of living and the struggle with nature, also won his sympathy for the Eskimos (and the Red Indians too). Imagination easily leads from the comfort of the warm feather-bed to the primitive state amongst the Eskimos. (*c*) " I know that " means I know from *Robinson Crusoe*. (*d*) The Eskimo ships were fitted out by analogy with the ships he had seen in Warnemünde. (*e*) We had never spoken to T. about the colour of the Eskimos. His supposition that they must have a differently coloured skin because they live in a land with a different climate is proof of a considerable capacity for productive, logical thinking. And does not blue fit in admirably with cold ! One would rather expect a child to come to the conclusion that Eskimos are white, because of the ice and snow of the polar regions. That would be easy to understand, but rather trivial. But blue is the colour of inward cold and frost. We may be accused of overestimating T's performance when we claim that what Goethe calls the " sensory and moral effect of colour " has here played its part. But how else is the choice to be explained ? It cannot have happened purely fortuitously, for T. is expressly seeking a connection between temperature and colour. T. can scarcely have heard that people go blue with cold, and he himself has always only gone red, so this experience would only cause him to choose red as the Eskimo colour.

67

10.5.26. Morning.

T. : (pointing to a parcel on a table) " What is there ? "

M. : " Baby-clothes."

T. : " Where did it come from ? "

M. : " Auntie L. borrowed it from us when she was expecting E–A. (the name of Auntie L's child, which T. had visited when it was a few weeks old)."

T. : " How did you know that E–A. was coming ? "

M. : " When children are coming you can notice it in their mothers, who get stouter because the children are growing inside them."

Discussion.—Here another perfectly natural opportunity arose to say a few words about the origin of children. As T. had visited the baby in question and become very fond of it, a friendly and serious feeling of attraction was spread over the whole complex of the idea. T. accepts the information given as something perfectly natural and does not spend any time in pondering over it.

68

27.5.26. Evening in bed.

J. : " Where do shop-assistants live ? " (*a*).

M. : " They live with their parents."

J. : " They have homes and live there with their Papas and Mamas. Have they any children too ? " (*b*).

M. : " Yes, many of them have children."

J. : " Yes, now I know."

Discussion.—What causes J. to speak about shop-assistants ? It can hardly be explained by association. (*a*) J's inquiry as to how they live may perhaps be connected with the fact that he has never seen in the shops any rooms fitted up for living in. (*b*) J. transposes what he hears into a more concrete form : in place of parents we get papas and mamas. Perhaps the question about children is asked without any reference to the shop-assistants and is produced associatively by the mention of papas and mamas.

69

1.6.26. M. and the children have gone to Warnemünde and are staying there till the end of August. To-day M. is writing a letter to F. and the children are helping her. M. was to write down everything. But at times they slip out of the atmosphere of letter-writing into the ordinary conventional tone.

T. : " Dear Papa, we had a safe journey here."

J. : " The boys (of the hotel proprietor) brought our things all right. Dear Papa, we have fine beds, we have plenty of space in each room " (a hint for Papa).

T. : " What will Papa think ? " (a).

J. : " He'll think we're boys from Warnemünde." (b).

T. : " But we're from Rostock." (c).

J. : " No, if you're gone away, then you're from Warnemünde." (d).

T. : " If Mama writes ' from Warnemünde' it's just the same as German." (e).

J. : " We saw the train going to Rostock, it could have waited till we came and went in it, then Papa would ask ' Where have you come from ? ' We'll say we've come from Warnemünde." (f).

T. : " We all send love and kisses." (g).

J. : " Let us draw B's (proprietor) house, or else Papa won't know where we are." (h).

T. : " Yes he will." (A house and people are sketched). " Mama, you are so small because we are so far away." (j).

Discussion.—At (a) the dialogue no longer connected with the letter begins and we only return to the subject at issue, the letter to F., at (g). The dialogue (a, b, c, d) between T. and J. reveals the difficulty the children experience in determining their relation to Rostock, where they live, and to Warnemünde, where they are on holiday, J. thinks the nationality of the new place has to be assumed. He does not succeed in ending the abstract formulation of the case which begins with the hypothetical " if you've gone away ", but instead he goes into a conclusion for the special case " then you're from Warnemünde ". (e) To an outsider this sentence must of necessity be incomprehensible. In Warnemünde the children hear much more Low German (Plattdeutsch) than in Rostock. T. now wants to express that even though Low German is spoken in Warnemünde, yet, since it can be understood, it is as good as German. So even in Warnemünde one can still be a German and therefore a Rostocker. The conversation takes a new turn at (*f*). J. has been made adventurous by the journey to Warnemünde and would like to travel back to Rostock and surprise F. (*h*) J. has by no means unbounded confidence in the written word : it would he thinks be better to draw the house itself where they are staying, so that F. may get a true impression of it. (*j*) We cannot say definitely what T. means. It is connected with his experience that people a great distance away look smaller : the smallness of the figure which represents M. in the drawing is connected with the idea of the great distance separating Warnemünde from Rostock in the eyes of F., for whom the sketch is intended. It illustrates and symbolizes this distance all in one.

70

3.6.26. Morning in bed. Character play.
M. : " Who are you ? "
J. : " We are elves ." (*a*).
M. : " What are you doing ? "
J. : " We've been in the forest."
M. : " What did you do there ? "
J. : " I chopped down some trees." (*b*).
T. : " I sat on a tree and did gym. and showed the others all kinds of things." (*c*).
J. : " We are witches too, we catch children and roast them." (*d*).

Discussion.—(*a, b, d*) J. is not consistent in his part as an elf, for chopping down trees is not the right occupation for elves. His temperament carries him away. Thus he goes on to play a wild witch, who catches and eats children. (*c*) T's activities as an elf run along more peaceful lines.

71

4.6.26. Morning in bed.
M. : " What did you dream, Theodor ? "
T. : " I dreamt that I wanted to buy a black mask and had no money, so I cut off the buttons from your fur-coat and that was my money." (*a*).

M. : " And what did you dream, Julius ? "

J. : " I dreamt that there'll be storm and lightning and thunder to-morrow and I said to the thunder : You must thunder everything down." (b).

Discussion.—(a) It is highly probable that T. did really dream this. The children liked to dress up and occasionally masks were used. Buttons and other round flat objects were treated as coins. We have to do with a wish dream in which in order to realize the wish an action is performed which would scarcely have been undertaken under the criticism of waking consciousness. (b) J. does not relate a dream, but makes up something on the spur of the moment, so as not to be behind his elder brother. The very fact that he claims to have dreamt what will happen to-morrow is against the genuineness of his account. The whole is rather a wish, and this wish again is characteristic of J. He wants things to be boisterous, with storm and thunder and lightning, and the words addressed to the thunder " You must thunder everything down " are lapidary.

72

5.6.26.   Morning in bed.

J. : " If we only get a baby to-morrow ! " (a).

T. : " But it must be a little boy, a little sister is not as rough as we, we can't play with her." (b).

J. : " You have to carry a baby and stroke it, you have to touch it very gently, not so roughly." (c).

T. : " I can't do that." (d).

Discussion.—(a) The desire to have a brother was frequently expressed by the children, and with special force whenever they had seen a baby at a friend's house. (b) This special wish about the sex of the desired baby is quite easy to understand. Compare the remarks in conversation 14, where girls are only esteemed as playmates if they are rough like boys. (c) J's remarks about how to treat a baby are charming. How touching is T's confession that he feels incapable of handling it as tenderly as J. demands.

73

5.6.26. Afternoon.

T. : " Apes are like a kind of human being, their mother looks in their hair just like our Mama (!) and they rock just like humans and have hands just like men." (*a*).

F. : " Who told you that ? "

T. : " Why, there are monkeys at Barnstorf." (i.e. I've seen and proved it for myself there.) (*b*).

J. : " And they jump on the rocking-horse and do silly things." (*c*).

Discussion.—(*a*) This statement shows splendid observation of monkeys' behaviour and also a most accurate independent drawing of analogies between the conduct of man and animals. Note what in monkeys appeared to him as similar to human beings ; we draw special attention to his noting the fact that they have " hands like men ". We have never drawn T's attention to this similarity, nor is it probable that it came from any outside source. The question was expressly asked by F. immediately afterwards, but denied (*b*) by referring to T's own (frequent) observations of the thing itself. (Once when we were standing in front of the chimpanzee's cage in the Berlin Zoo, a teacher with a class of children came along. One of the huge creatures advanced from the background and a twelve-year-old boy called out " There's a black ". The anthropoid had at once been taken for a negro. Perhaps to unprejudiced children the similarity between apes and men appears greater than it does to adults). (*c*) The animals are especially attractive to J. because they do silly things —at least according to his view. It is a question of recognizing one's own character in another living creature and being delighted at finding it there. J's remark is not intended as a contribution to the theme of similarity to human beings.

74

6.6.26. Morning in bed.

T. : " Mama, tell us about America."

M. : (Tells, as she has done on several previous occasions,

the story of the discovery of America in a form the children can understand.)

T. : " And were the black people already there ? " (a).

M. : " No, they were brought from Africa in ships by the whites."

J. : " If they had known, then they'd have disguised themselves, and a policeman ought to have come and arrested them." (b).

T. : " Were the black people always black ? " (c).

M. : " Yes."

T. : " And the whites ? " (d).

M. : " They were always white."

J. : " And they (the blacks) ought to have got a motor car and run over them (the whites) and got guns and shot them." (e).

T. : " Did the black people go back to Africa ? " (f).

M. : " No, they got accustomed to America."

T. : " Mama, there must be cannons, to shoot at the ice." (g).

M. : " Yes, when ice is causing a flood, it is shot at with cannon."

T. : " Or else the ice gets higher and higher (h). Mama, was Berlin discovered too ? " (j).

M. : " Berlin was built. Before that the land where Berlin now stands was discovered."

Discussion.—(a) The children had heard of slavery and its abolition. T's question is an attempt to touch on this theme. (b, e) How quickly childish indignation rises against the evil of slavery. Disguise, policeman, arrest, and then J's proposals continue, without being interrupted by the dialogue which M. and T. still carry on. It is perseveration. He lets the blacks give the whites a dreadful time. (c, d) T. has once again sought information whether the blacks and whites have always had skins of those colours. The return of the blacks to Africa (f) would indeed have been the best solution to a problem which causes America and the negroes so much suffering. The child finds this solution in all simplicity, or at least hints at it in his question. (g) Now the conversation takes an entirely new turn. The shooting, of which J. has been speaking, brings cannon into T's mind, but he will only use them for peaceful purposes (*h*). (*j*) The discovery complex still perseverates in T., it is impossible to say why at this point he chooses Berlin as an object to be discovered.

75

7.6.26. Morning.

M. : " Theodor, you must not strike ; that is assault, and assault is a punishable offence."

T. : " Was David punished because he hit Goliath ? " (*a*).

M. : " No. But you know David fought with Goliath."

T. : " And then David became Emperor." (*b*).

M. : " David became king."

T. : " No, he must have become Emperor." (*c*).

M. : " Julius, tell me something."

J. : " We were shoremen, we were eating on the shore. You must tell us when we have to come home. When we are shoremen, we go into the water." (*d*).

M. : " What else do you do ? "

J. : " I don't know."

Discussion.—(*a*) T. had pushed Auntie O., and therefore M. gave the above warning half in fun and half seriously. The practical application of the David-Goliath case comes as a surprise. (*b*, *c*) In fairy tales the Emperor is the highest person, and so also for T., who therefore makes David an Emperor and persists in his opinion in spite of M. (*d*) Shoremen, an appropriate new creation of J., which he constantly used.

76

8.6.26. Evening in bed.

J. : " Elli ran away from me. Did you ever see such a girl ? Let's send Elli away." (*a*).

T. : " In a parcel." (*b*).

J. : " Yes, in a parcel, we'll make a hole in it." (*c*).

T. : " A big hole like this " (indicates with his hands.) (*d*).

M. : " What is the hole for ? "

J. : " For Elli to get air, or else she may suffocate. Elli doesn't know that one has to stay with children." (*e*).

T. : " Once when she was with us she went out and said : ' I'll be back in a minute,' and she didn't come back." (*f*).

J. : " Then Grannie came, she didn't go out, she stayed with us." (*g*).

M. : " Theodor, have you done anything naughty ? "

T. : " I ran away from Grannie and went to the water, but not close to. I thought there were some cockchafers there but they had been washed away by the water." (*h*).

M. : " You must not run away from Grannie. Her legs are stiff and she can't run after you. Children must not go near the water alone."

T. : " We only wanted to see how a ship was being tugged ashore and then a boy threw sand at us and so I threw sand at him." (*j*).

M. : " It is better to go away from children who throw sand."

T. : " But we were only just looking how the ship was pulled ashore (*k*). Mama, does the stomach grind (i.e. digest) milk too ? " (*e*).

M. : " Yes, the stomach digests milk too. Milk contains a great deal of water as well as fat."

T. : " Why is there water in milk ? "

M. : " All drinks contain water."

J. : " What's in Berni (conv. 55) is really true, isn't it ? " (*m*).

T. : " But it says in Berni that there was an old woman who had red eyes, her fingers were like claws, she had a lot of animals, sparrows too."

J. : " When a witch jumps over a human being and says ' hocuspocus ' then the human being is turned into a tiger." (*n*).

M. : " There aren't any witches."

J. : " There are witches in fairy tales, but really there aren't any witches."

M. : " Julius, what will you be called when you are grown up, will you be called Theodor then ? " (Test connected with conversation 56.)

J. : " I will be called Herr Professor Katz and Theodor will be called Frau Professor Katz : I shall marry Theodor, then he will be my son and I'll marry you and Auntie O. too, then I shall have two wives." (*o*).

M. : " Julius, have you done anything wrong to-day ? "

J. : " No, only good."

T. : " Where did the Great War begin, here in Rostock ? " (*p*).

M. : " The Great War began on the frontier between Russia and Germany."

T. : " Where did the Great War end ? "

M. : " The Great War ended in France."

T. : " And was that the very end ? "

M. : " Yes, in France."

Discussion.—(*a*) J. is annoyed that E. went away from him, she must be sent back to her parents. (*b, c, d, e*) Considerations as to the best means of sending back E. T. and J. think people can be sent through the post, as they once saw a dog sent. (*f, g*) Further complaints about E., whose conduct is contrasted with that of Grannie. (*h, j, k*) Previously T. had been very obedient to our refusal to allow him to go near the water. But at this time the shore was too attractive because of the cockchafers to be found there, and in addition there was a ship at a point on the coast where ships very rarely came. The transition to (*l*) and from (*l*) to (*m*) is not clear. (*n*) Whether this knowledge was derived from the servants, or is due to imagination, we cannot say. (*o*) Here we have a jumble of serious and joking statements. J. may believe that he will later on be F., but all the rest is poured wildly out just as chance combines to connect the persons cropping up in his mind. (*p*) T. believes that his native town must be the head of everything, even to the extent that the Great War must have begun there.

77

9.6.26. Afternoon. F. is visiting M. and the children in Warnemünde.

F. : " Do you know what kind of an animal we have now at the Institute ? "

J. : " The monkey ! "

F. : " No, we have a little dog."

J. : " The monkey would have taken all the books and

made a mess of everything. If you had picked up a book he would have taken it away from you."

F. : " What else would he do ? "

J. : " Then he might sit at your writing desk and type. If the monkey types, you won't need to type."

Discussion.—A monkey for experimental purposes was expected in the animal psychology department of the Institute. The children were looking forward to the day of its arrival with the greatest impatience. This breaks out when F. asks the first question. J. thinks only of the monkey, and paying no attention to F's correction, he imagines what confusion the monkey will cause in the Institute. After seeing the monkeys in the Zoo he believes the animal will be so human that it will be able to use the typewriter.

78

9.6.26. Afternoon. M. is playing " man and wife " with J. J. brings some stuffed animals.

M. : " It will be very nice to have animals in the stable ; this cat for instance can catch mice."

J. : " No, she mustn't catch our mice, or else we won't have any mice." (He is probably thinking of the white mice at the Institute, with which he always liked to play.) " She mustn't catch our dog either. Here, wife, we have a windmill, coloured chalk, a book." (J. rings.)

T. : " You can ring as much as you like. I want to rest now, you ragged beggar." (*a*).

J. : " I'm another man now." (*b*).

T. : " What do you want, ragged old beggar ? " (*c*).

J. : " May your carcase rot." (*d*).

M. : " No, you mustn't say things like that."

Discussion.—In character plays J. was always liable, as here, to forget completely to keep up his part. (*a, b, c, d*) The conversation which develops between the two children is distinguished by a rudeness of expression derived from the puppet plays and Punch and Judy.

79

9.6.26. Evening in bed.

T. : " How does the earth turn ? " (*a*).

M. : " The earth turns like a ball. The side turned towards the sun has day, the other side has night."

T. : " And in the Canary Isles ? " (*b*).

M. : " When the Canary Isles are turned towards the sun it is day there, otherwise it is night."

T. : " Is Gehlsdorf an island ? " (*c*).

M. : " No, Gehlsdorf is a peninsula, because we can get from Rostock to Gehlsdorf on foot. An island is entirely surrounded by water."

T. : " How do you get to Gehlsdorf ? " (*d*).

M. : " Past the White Cross."

T. : " Sometime I want to walk to Gehlsdorf." (*e*).

M. : " Yes, you could do that now."

T. : " When you go to Copenhagen, do you go past an island ? " (*f*).

M. : " Yes."

Discussion.—Throughout a geographical conversation. (*a*) T. has previously learned that the earth revolves, now he wants further details. (*b*) The general statement must now be exemplified in the Canary Isles. But why there? Because they are mentioned in the beloved *Robinson Crusoe*. (*c*) The question is justified because up to then T. had always gone to Gehlsdorf on the ferry across the Warnow. (*d, e*) Utterances caused by the desire to make voyages of exploration. (*f*) T. attempts here to apply what he has just learned to the special case of the journey to Denmark. This short dialogue is noteworthy for the beauty of its logical development by T.

80

10.6.26. Forenoon, immediately after Puss in Boots has been read aloud.

T. : " Was the King discovered too ? "

M. : " No, the King was elected."

T. : " Was Berlin discovered ? "

M. : " No, Berlin was built by the people who had settled there."

L

Discussion.—T. is still not clear about the meaning of " discover " and indeed it is not easy. So it is easy to understand why T. uses it when he wants to ask about the origin of the king. The information (in conv. 74) that Berlin was not discovered, was not sufficient.

81

12.6.26. After dinner. The children are to sleep as usual, J. in his bed, T. on the sofa (at the seaside). J. says that to-day he would prefer to sleep with his brother on the sofa. If he did so, of course neither would go to sleep, but they would only disturb each other and get into mischief.

J. : " I want to sleep with Theodor on the sofa."

M. : " Don't you love me any more then, that you don't want to sleep near me ? " (J's bed stood near his mother's.)

J. : " I love Theodor most." (a).

M. : " Then sleep with Theodor, but I shall sleep in both beds."

J. : " I want to sleep with T. so that you can get some rest." (b).

G. : " Do you want to sleep with me ? "

J. : " No, you must have rest, Grannie, and Mama must have rest. Mama can lie in two beds also." (c).

Discussion.—(a) The deciding factor in J's expression of his desire, is the amusement he sees in prospect if he may be together with his brother on the sofa. He does not desire in the least to sleep on the sofa, but to play there as he has done so often. True he says " sleep " and it may be that at the moment he means it, but the only explanation of his behaviour is provided by the play impulse which is in the background of his consciousness. Now he suddenly discovers that he loves T. most ; it is possible that he believes this too for the moment, but in reality it is only a disguise of the play impulse. He is not in the least disconcerted, but can give other reasons for his desire—how touching is his anxiety about the rest of M. (b) and G. (c) although at other times very little of this is to be observed. We have here a model example of the case where a motive other than the true one is given for behaviour, because the true motive could not withstand criticism, whilst the motive advanced has more prospect of being admitted by the people concerned. In the case at issue the fictitious nature even lets J. appear in a heroic light. No psychoanalysis is needed to see through J., indeed we do not doubt that he would laughingly have admitted the true motive had we asked him outright. It is worthy of special notice that we can see as clearly as possible the will to disguise motives even in a child not quite four years old.

82

12.6.26. Evening in bed.

T. : " Julius, why didn't you see us to-day ? (i.e. when T and M. went past the tram in which you and G. were sitting)."

J. : " I did see you." (a).

T. : " No."

J. : " I don't know, I saw a boy in a red sweater, like you, and a lady with a hat and blouse like Mama. The lady came to our table and took eggs and bread and butter from the rucksack and then we had a meal." (b).

T. : " But that was Mama."

J. : " Mama, was it you ? " (c).

M. : " Yes, it was I."

J. : " That was at the inn." (d).

T. : " No, that wasn't at the inn, we didn't see any pigs, and cows, and they are at the inn." (e).

M. : " Julius, if you get lost and you are asked where you live and what your name is, what will you say ? "

J. : " I am called Julius Gregor Katz."

M. : " And where do you live ? "

J. : " In Kaiser-Wilhelm-Platz." (f).

M. : " Don't you live in Moltkestrasse any more ? "

J. : " Yes, in Moltkestrasse."

M. : " What number ? "

J. : " What number ? "

M. : " Number thirteen."

J. : " Thirteen."

M. : " And where do you live in Warnemünde ? "

J. : " At B's."

M. : " Which street ? "

J. : " I don't know."

M. : " Anastasiastrasse."

J. : " Anastasiastrasse." (Repeats it several times). " What number ? "

M. : " Number fourteen."

J. : " Fourteen."

M. : (joking) " Then you'll say that you are loved."

J. : " Other people needn't know that, they love their own children." (g).

M. : " But you can perhaps say that you are loved."

J. : " No, because they don't know that I'm Julius and they'll say we didn't love you ; I don't love them either." (h).

Discussion.—(a) The question whether J. saw M. and T. from the tram is answered in the affirmative, but circumstances made it impossible and T. quite correctly disputes the reply. The remarks (b) are very remarkable. It appears that J. has not connected the question with meeting on the way, but with being together at the inn for the meal. The stay at the inn lasted about two hours, then all set out home, M. and T. on foot, J. and G. by tram. It is at once remarkable in itself that J. should connect the question of having seen M. and T. with the inn, for if an adult who has been in the company of close relatives for several hours, were asked whether he had seen them, he would certainly not understand the question as referring to the time spent together, but to some other meeting where it would have been quite possible to miss seeing each other. But it is still more remarkable that J. describes the clothing of M. and T. quite correctly, but does not immediately identify the lady and the boy in his mind as M. and T. J. reveals himself so open to suggestion on this point, that he falsifies the whole structure of obvious experiences and changes M. and his brother into strangers, or at least lets them be changed. (c) What does he really believe in his heart of hearts ? That he was with strangers ? Probably not. J. gets into a state hovering between belief and doubt, a state extremely difficult to characterize and one which adults can never fully experience. This much is clear from this experience, that the four year old child's conception of reality is still completely different from that of the adult. It is so easy to overlook the gulf between the two conceptions, because the child's language, in a four year old approximately the same as an adult's, usually conceals these things rather than reveals them. (d) J's assumption that it was in the inn is correct and confirms our view that J. was referring to the stay there. From T's statement that it was not at the inn we see that he had a conception of the inn which we had not suspected till then. At this inn there were pigs and cows, and when we were there we went as a rule to look at these animals. It appears now that T. only spoke about the inn with reference to the most important things living there, i.e. the animals. The whole farm as such, together with the public rooms, had not been understood as " inn ". (f) The Kaiser-Wilhelm-Platz is in the immediate vicinity of our house in Rostock, and has made a greater impression on J. than the house itself. (g) J. understands that M. is only joking, but he takes it more seriously than T. would do ; T. only smiles. (h) An explanation very much to the point. The form " loved " is suggested to him by the same form in M's preceding remark.

83

13.6.26. Afternoon. T. leans lovingly against M.
M. : " Well, what about your love ? "
T. : " I love Papa a little more than you, because you know I'll be a Papa too, so I must love Papa more."

Discussion.—Strange logic is revealed by this remark. It may be that T. at the moment really has warmer feelings towards F., and that he puts forward the fact, that he will later on be a father, in order not to hurt M. But it may also be that T. deduces from his later fatherhood that he *must* love F. more. It is scarcely possible to decide between these alternatives.

84

17.6.26. Afternoon.
J. : " We have caught some cockchafers."
F. : " Where are they ? "
J. : " We put him in the grass in the garden."
F. : " Why, will he eat grass ? "
J. : " If he eats leaves, he'll eat grass too." (*a*).
F. : " Did you see the cockchafer's wife too ? "
J. : " Yes, she's on the shore." (*b*).

Discussion.—(*a*) Quite a good conclusion even though not accurate in fact. (*b*) J. takes F's joking question seriously. It is quite possible that at the moment he is convinced he has seen the cockchafer's wife on the shore.

85

18.6.26. Afternoon on the shore.
J. : (pointing to a two-year-old child) " I'd like to have a child like that." (*a*).
F. : " Why should you like a child like that ? "
J. : " To play baby with it." (*b*).
F. : " Would you like a little brother or a little sister ? "
J. : " A little brother."
F. : " Why not a sister ? "
J. : " Well, we are both boys and so it must be a boy too. When we play policemen, then it (the sister) will cry Mama, Mama, and that won't do." (*c*).

Discussion.—(*a*) As both children had often expressed the wish for a little baby we thought at first that J's remark was to be understood in this sense. But (*b*) showed that J. is thinking more of playing baby with the child, just as he himself must often be the baby when playing with T. The baby that F. presents to J. must be a boy (*c*) so that it can take part in the boys' boisterous games.

86

20.6.26. Forenoon.
M. : " You must not come in and disturb us when I have visitors."

T.: " Why not, I only want to hear what you are talking about." (a).

M.: " When grown-ups talk, children don't understand and so they need not listen."

T.: " But I do understand that a maid is untidy and tells lies." (b).

M.: " You see, the lady said how wrong it is when one tells lies. You don't tell lies, do you."

T.: " No, Mama, but I did tell two lies." (c).

M.: " That is very bad. When was it ? "

T.: " Once I climbed through the window (ground floor flat in Warnemünde) and when Auntie O. asked me I said I hadn't." (d).

M.: " Why did you not tell Auntie O. that you had come in through the window ? "

T.: (proudly) " No, I told a lie."

M.: " You must always have the courage to tell the truth."

Discussion.—(a) T. regards himself as perfectly entitled to take part in the conversations of adults who visit us. We first noticed about this time that T. was showing interest in conversations of the parents, either between themselves or with other adults. We had not suspected this because the subjects discussed did not immediately concern him, but about this time he began to break in with questions which showed that he had been following the course of conversation. So from that point onwards we had to exercise care in discussing affairs which he was not to hear. Usually children hear, in families, too much about things which ought to remain unknown to them, because it is believed they will not listen to conversations which have no direct interest for them. (b) This had actually been the subject of the conversation. (c) Setting up the general principle that one ought not to tell lies causes T. to confess with pride that he has lied twice. " Twice " probably means here " twice recently ", although, as it subsequently appears, it was really only once. In defence of T's honour we can state that he really does not tell lies and we have never caught him in the act of lying. (d) T. did not get on very well with Auntie O. He was always on the defensive against her, and so perhaps he regards a lie as a permissible weapon in the circumstances, just as a schoolboy regards (or regarded ?) a lie as a permissible means of opposing his teacher whereas he detests untruthfulness in classmates and parents. T. probably was afraid that Auntie O. would punish him, and so he did not summon up courage enough to tell the truth. His parents did not punish him when he confessed his misdemeanours to them, but instructed him how he must do better in future. (*e*) This statement means probably " I could have told the truth then to Auntie O, but I didn't, and now, as a brave boy I am ready to take the consequences of my action."

87

21.6.26. Morning.

M. : " Auntie N. sends her love. You are to order fine weather and then her children will come and visit you."

T. : " How shall I order fine weather ? "

M. : " Just think."

T. : " I know. Let's make a kite and tie a letter to it, then we'll send the kite up ; Nature is up there, and the letter will be read and then we've ordered fine weather."

Discussion.—T. takes the joking expression seriously and considers how to solve the problem. The solution he provides is by no means bad.

88

22.6.26. Evening.

T. : " Mama, I want to be a dustman." (*a*).

M. : " Why do you want to be a dustman ? "

T. : " Then I can dig." (*b*).

J. : " Only little children say dustman, grown-ups say duster." (*c*).

T. : " Mama, Hans S. throws sand at us." (*d*).

M. : " I'll tell him not to do it."

J. : " Let's throw sand at him, then it will get in his eyes and he'll know about it." (*e*).

Discussion.—(*a, b*) The motive for the new choice of profession is clear. He has been so delighted digging in the sand by the sea, that he would like to become a dustman in order to exercise his talents in this direction. (*c*) J. regards dustman as equivalent to duster, a mistake which shows what misconceptions children have about words which sound somewhat alike. (*d, e*) From the point of view of character it is interesting to note the different attitudes adopted by the two brothers to the actions of a third person. T. seeks M's assistance whereas J. is ready to put up an energetic defence himself.

89

22.6.26. Evening. A married couple, friends of ours, have come to go for a walk with M.

J. : " Mama, why are you going out ? "

M. : " I am going a little way with Auntie and Uncle B., they've been sitting in the house all day and must have some fresh air."

J. : " Well, they've walked here so they've had some fresh air."

Discussion.—J. takes M's reason for the walk literally and then is quite right in raising his objection in order to prevent M. from leaving him.

90.

28.6.26. Midday at table. T. has been taking part for some time in gymnastics for children, and is becoming quite skilful.

F. : " Theodor, some day you'll be a clever gymnast."

T. : " No, I don't want to be a gymnast, I want to be a diver. On Sundays when I'm not diving I'll do gymnastics, and sometimes in the evening when I'm not diving."

Discussion.—T. had understood F. to mean that he should adopt gymnastics as his profession. He declines. He is now turning to a new profession, never mentioned previously, the diving profession, obviously under the influence of his experience in Warnemünde. There he saw a diving ship and the diver himself in his wonderful diving-suit and after that he was never tired of hearing about a diver's activities. So he won't become a gymnast, but, as a relaxation from his professional work he will do a little gymnastics on Sundays and in the evening when it is too dark to dive. We should also like to mention that the ideal of becoming a diver persisted an extremely long time.

91

30.6.26. Afternoon.

F. : " What would you like for your birthday ? "

J. : " A toffee heart and some nut-toffee. A little wooden pony that will rock to and fro."

F. : " What colour shall it be ? "

J. : " Green."

F. : " And what else ? "

J. : " White."

F. : " What else do you want ? "

J. : " A forest ? "

F. : " A real one ? "

J. : " No, a wooden one."

F. : " What else ? "

J. : " A train and rails and a ship, and a sailor who can row."

F. : " What else ? "

J. : " Do you know what I want too ? "

F. : " Well ? "

J. : " A motor car so that children can get in, all children."

F. : " A motor car."

J. : " When you pedal it goes. One for me and one for Theodor."

F. : " And have you any other wishes ? "

J. : " A wooden snail. A hunting dog and huntsmen, not living."

Discussion.—What is the heart's desire of a four-year-old child ? These birthday wishes betray it to us. Many of the things J. enumerates have more individual value, but still who, as a child, would not have been delighted with this array of sweets and toys ? It is not claimed that

J. mentions the wishes in a well-arranged order, so that the most important come first. Here and there F's encouragement was necessary to cause J. to express further wishes. Such conversations can contribute towards giving us an insight into the scale of values in the life of the child at various ages.

92

1.7.26. Night, before going to sleep.
T. : " Mama, I can scarcely express how much I love you, but even less how much I love Papa."
J. : " Mama, I love you like all the towns."
M. : " And papa ? "
J. : " I love Papa like all the towns, too."

Discussion.—We could notice how occasionally T. was overcome by the consciousness of his boundless fondness for his parents. How beautiful is this declaration of love to the parents, in all its touching helplessness. J. does not want to lag behind T., but he would scarcely have made such a declaration spontaneously. The standard of his love is rather unusual, he treats M. and F. both alike.

93

2.7.26. At supper.
M. : " Theodor, would you like an egg ? "
T. : " Yes, and perhaps Julius too."
M. : " Would you like an egg, Julius ? "
J. : " No, meat."
T. : " Like a tiger."

Discussion.—A short conversation characterizing the previously mentioned tastes of T. and J. T's last remark is said in all seriousness.

94

3.7.26. After the meal.
J. : " When I am a captain I'll take you all on my ship because you fed me so well when I was small. Theodor will then be a diver ; then I'll pull him up high with a rope."

Discussion.—Only a short monologue but so revealing characterologically that it must be included. Good food is a very important affair to a four-year-old child, and especially important to a boy with such a healthy appetite as J. develops at the seaside. He will not forget those who have provided him with such good food, and as a reward they are all to travel on the ship of which he is captain. The profession of ship's captain is the first one J. kept for any length of time. Very pretty is the idea of the two brothers working in common in their later life as captain and diver.

95

4.7.26. Afternoon. J. has a slight sore throat and is kept in bed with a poultice round his throat.

J. : " I must be well for my birthday (6.7) or else the children will come and I'll be ill and there'll be lots of fine things, that won't do." (*a*).

F. : " Yes, I'll soon make you well again."

J. : " We'll put ointment on and make a poultice." (*b*).

F. : " Yes, we'll do that."

J. : " What do you think I'll get for my birthday ? I'd like to have so much that the table *nearly* breaks ; it mustn't crack or else Frau B. (the landlady) will come and be cross with us (*c*). Do you know what goats do when they are glad ? Goats say meh. So do lambs, they're sheep too." (*d*).

F. : " What do cows say when they're glad ? "

J. : " They say moo."

F. : " And how are fish glad ? "

J. : " Fish aren't glad, they've got no voice you know." (*e*).

F. : " And how are human beings glad ? "

J. : " Like this, hahaha."

F. : " Yes, humans are glad like that.—Now I'll tell you a story about Princess Zizibe."

T. (anxiously) " Is it a terrible story ? "

F. : " No, it isn't terrible."

Discussion.—(*a*) J's birthday is on 6th July. Naturally there has been a great deal of talk about it in the last few days. J. is very concerned that he may still be ill on his birthday, but as there are to be so many fine things, that simply must not happen—just as if it were within mortal power to dismiss illness by order. Perhaps we may say a few words here about the reaction of children to illness and the doctor. We believe that this relation, at least with reference to medicine, may be designated as magical. Everything that can be classed as medicine is probably considered by the child as magical, which is acting immediately, not by stages. He believes in the doctor and his medicine, just as primitive man believes in a medicine man and his process of healing.[1] The medical man, " Uncle Doctor " really plays the part of the medicine man for the child. As can easily be demonstrated, in feverish illness children become very apathetic ; by such an illness they are temporarily thrown back several stages, maybe years, in their intellectual level. In infectious illnesses our children revealed a very marked need of rest, and usually asked for themselves to be put into bed. In illness children withdraw from society, a habit which may also be observed amongst gregarious animals. Usually our children displayed a touching patience when ill, they were indeed much more patient than any adult would have been. On this point doctors have told us of the astonishing patience with which children accommodate themselves to remaining sometimes for days or even weeks in some recumbent or uncomfortable position for orthopædic reasons. (b) J. here proposes himself that a poultice should be applied and that he should be treated with ointment. He believes that the ointment, which had once before cured his chapped skin, must have an effective healing action in every case. In the ointment (as in every medicine) there resides, so to speak, health itself, and this health can be incorporated in the human body by rubbing (or taking internally).[2] (c) Often we have

---

[1] With regard to ethnological parallel, read Th. W. Danzel, *Magie und Geheimwissenschaft in ihrer Bedeutung für Kultur und Kulturgeschichte*, Stuttgart, 1924.

[2] The uneducated adult has usually a very similar idea of the curative effect of medicine.

said jokingly, that on such and such a person's birthday there were so many presents that the table broke. J., too, would like to have so many presents that the table *almost* breaks, but not quite, so that the landlady shall not make any fuss, for she is the authority for which he has so much respect that he even consents to rest in bed every afternoon. (*d*) Now we have some very interesting considerations of how various animals make it known that they are glad. Lambs, as little sheep, are particularly singled out by J., a thing which an adult would not do, but lambs represent to the children something quite novel as compared to sheep. But then J. confesses that after all they, too, are sheep and so will show they are glad in the same way that sheep do. (*e*) Surprisingly we learn that fishes are never glad because they have no voice, or we might also say it is not really surprising, for probably in children the expression of a sentiment coincides with that sentiment to a far greater extent than in adults.[1] We are inclined to believe that the man in the street also feels a much greater psychological unity between expression and the thing expressed, than does the reflecting psychologist. (*f*) T. does not want a terrible story ; here we note the influence of the psychological experience he has gained, that terrifying stories heard just before going to bed, tend to disturb him.

96

5.7.26. On the beach at Warnemünde.
T. : " Mama, I'd rather be in Rostock." (*a*).
J. : " Don't you like being at Warnemünde ? "
T. : " No, it's nicer in Rostock, it's hot there and we get as black as niggers there." (*b*).
M. : " Julius, do you like being at Warnemünde ? "
J. : " Yes."
M. : " Why do you like being in Warnemünde so much ? "
J. : " There's sand here and sun, and *everything* here is fine." (*c*).
M. : " Shall we go back to Rostock, soon ? "
J. : " No, there's no sand there, you know."

[1] " The chair can't laugh of course, he's got no teeth." (Stern, p. 346.)

Discussion.—When F. visited Warnemünde from Rostock, he frequently mentioned that it was much cooler on the beach in Warnemünde than in the grilling town. This may be considered as the cause of T's preference (*a*) for Rostock. His ideal is, although he is already very sunburned, to get as black as a nigger (*b*). (*c*) J. has no feeling for this romantic attitude, but would prefer to stay in Warnemünde, where everything seems bright and happy.

97

6.7.26. The children are playing with two boys of 10 and 12 years old. T. has quickly struck up a friendship with Hans-Borchardt the elder. In the course of their play the name " Appelschnut " is mentioned.

J. : " That's Appelschnut. Appelschnut is silly, she wanted to reach the sun, she'd have to walk for a thousand years." (*a*).

T. : " Then she'd be old (*b*). You're called Hans-Borchardt, and your brother ? " (*c*).

H. B. : " My brother's name is Rolf."

T. : " Those are nice names, I like them, and I am called Wilhelm Theodor Katz, and what is my Papa's name ? " (*d*).

H. B. : " I don't know."

Discussion.—(*a*) Appelschnut appears to have made an impression on both boys with her naïveté, which is interpreted by them as foolishness. In Conversation 34, T. criticized her conduct, and now the younger brother is doing the same. The estimate of the distance of the sun in years must have come from adults, as J. has of course no proper idea of his own estimate. (*b*) The semi-ironical remark of T. is quite remarkable. (*c, d*) The interest in the names of the two new playmates is occasioned by interest in the playmates themselves, as the game was already well under way. For the child, just as for primitive man, the name is an essential part of the person. T. transfers his feelings to the bearers of the names to the names themselves. He considers it his duty to mention his own name then, just as in any official introduction. What sweet simplicity for T. to believe that everyone must of course know his father's name.

98

9.7.26. Early morning.

J. : " I am now a clown, and will paint my fingers red. Mama, write a notice that my name is now Karl, for a clown can't be called Julius of course. Julius is a child's name, isn't it ? and when I get to the station then the ticket-collector will think I'm a clown."

Discussion.—Once more a monologue, but so revealing for J's thought process and in itself so charming, that it deserves a place here. The children had visited a Punch and Judy show, where the clown above all had delighted them. J. would now like to be a clown himself, and as a sign of his new dignity he will paint his fingers red. Why is M. to write a notice that he is now called Karl ? A clown of course can't be called Julius, for Julius is the name of little boys like himself, and belongs so to speak to the material group " little boys ". So the name is to be *written down*, because that is more definite and proof positive. It can be given to adults to read, and then they'll believe it. Furthermore J. thinks that when he gets to the station the ticket-collector will regard him as a clown because of his external appearance, and so the name must harmonize with this, or else he will be taken for Julius.

99

10.7.26. Evening before going to bed.

T. : " Mama, I shouldn't like to go to hell."

M. : " Who's been telling you about hell, Theodor ? "

T. : " Auntie O. said if we're naughty we'll go to hell and get roasted there."

M. : " There isn't any hell, people have only imagined such a thing in order to frighten others. When children run about a lot, people say the bogey man will come, but there isn't any bogey man, and there isn't any hell. You've no need to be afraid, you won't go to hell."

Discussion.—Once more a pedagogical masterpiece by a trained children's nurse. The child's terror proves its effect.

O. has probably never suspected what torment such stories about hell would cause the child. What defence has a child against such ideas? It has nothing to oppose to them, and cannot defend itself against them. The most serious thing is that the damage, once done, can only be very slowly repaired. Strong counter-suggestion, extending over a long period is necessary, in order to demolish a complex such as this hell-complex. Indeed it seems very doubtful whether a complete demolition is possible at all during childhood. And even if, as an adult, one ridicules such childish impressions, that does not mean that their effect is nullified and that they are thereby banished.

100

13.7.26. At supper.

M. : " Julius, eat your egg, or the hen will say she won't lay any more eggs for you."

J. : " And the cock ? " (a).

M. : " The cock will say, I shan't allow you to treat the eggs my wife lays like this."

J. : " And do his children lay eggs too ? " (b).

M. : " No, the children are too small yet."

T. : " But when the children grow up, they'll lay eggs too, won't they ? " (c).

M. : " Yes, when the chickens have grown up, they'll lay eggs. Theodor, do you think they'll all lay eggs ? "

T. : " No. The boy chickens won't lay any eggs, only the girls." (d).

Discussion.—(a) J. does not mean by his question to ask whether the cock will perhaps lay an egg for him instead of the hen, but he is asking " What will the cock say ? " i.e. not merely to this particular question, but in general. (b) We have the obvious step from the parents to the children. (c) This must be so, because young animals grow up, and he knows that grown-up creatures do lay eggs. (d) The inner reason why the " boy chickens " should lay no eggs is naturally quite unknown to T. To him egg-laying is merely an affair of the female of the species. The following conversation reveals how innocent T. still is in such matters.

M

101

15.7.26. The D. family, our former hosts in Warnemünde, had just had a baby, and our children were extremely interested.

T. : " Kurt D. thought he was going to be alone, but now there's a baby. Is it a little boy or a little girl ? "

F. : " How can you tell whether it is a girl or a boy ? "

T. : " At first I never know whether it is a boy or a girl, but later I can tell by the long hair." (a).

J. : " I am a human being." (b).

F. : " So you're a human being, are you ? "

J. : " Yes, of course, for I can speak. Animals can't speak, you know." (c).

Discussion.—(a) This charmingly naïve remark might reasonably appear in a humorous periodical. It is unnecessary to point out that it is genuine naïveté.[1] (b) A lapidary statement. Has J. only just discovered that he is a human being ? And what leads him to formulate his discovery just at this moment ? It is difficult to say. (c) His method of differentiation for homo sapiens is perfectly acceptable, if we take " speak " in its fullest sense.

102

17.7.26. Early morning.

T. : " Berni got a school outfit too for Christmas." (a).

M. : " Yes, you've already got everything, your satchel, slate, and lunch-tin."

T. : " And I've had a bag of sweets too." (b).

M. : " We can fill up the bag again."

T. : " No, I've had the bag full once, I don't need any more. I don't need to have again what I've already had once."

Discussion.—(a) Here, after a long interval, his good friend Berni appears once more. Berni has become the standard

---

[1] " The difference between boys and girls in Bubi's opinion consists principally in the different clothing and Christian names." Ernst and Gertrud Scupin, *Bubi im vierten bis sechsten Lebensjahr*, Leipzig, 1910, p. 170.

for many of the things that one may or may not do, should or should not do. For T., Berni was really the first boyish ideal, and was later supplanted in this position by *Robinson Crusoe*. (*b*) The bag of sweets was the most important thing and must not be forgotten. T's refusal to allow the bag to be refilled is thoroughly typical of his modest character which about this time was coming more and more into evidence.

103

19.7.26. Evening.
J. : " It's morning now where the negroes live." (*a*).
M. : " Yes, the negroes are just getting up and washing."
J. : " But it's no use the negroes washing, they remain black just the same." (*b*).
T. : " Does the sun make the negroes so black, or are negro children born black ? " (*c*).
F. : " They are black when they are born."
T. : " But they do get a little blacker with the sun, don't they ? " (*d*).
F. : " Yes, negro children are at first lighter coloured and then get darker."

Discussion.—(*a*) The children had been delighted when they heard that the antipodes have day when we have night and vice versa. The negroes were classed at once as antipodes ; probably the colour of their skin, which represents the opposite of day, played its part also. (*b*) A very natural idea, that when negroes wash it is due to a desire to get rid of the black colour, just as the children do when they wash. In other conversations about the colour of negroes' skin the idea had been put forward, that washing could actually have the result of making a negro white. The questions (*c*, *d*) are connected with remarks in previous conversations. T's experiences on the beach at Warnemünde make it impossible for him not to believe that the sun must exert a darkening influence in the ontogenetic sense even on the skin of negroes. We had no scruples in allowing him to continue in this belief.

104

20.7.26. Afternoon. T. and Auntie O. were at loggerheads.

T. : " Auntie M. (the head mistress of the Kindergarten which T. formerly attended) ought to have made you stand in a corner."

O. : " Auntie M. didn't make me stand in a corner, it was you, you."

T. : " But only for a moment, and if I was (he means had been) big and strong I'd have hit Auntie M."

Discussion.—T. feels injured and descends to a type of punishment for Auntie O., which is very commonly used in the circles in which T. learned it. It is unwise of Auntie O. to react as she does to T's remarks, which admittedly are very improper. She reminds him of a punishment the form of which must have hurt T. very much. This we may see from the fact that the memory of the punishment has lingered so long and from the feelings which T. had when he was made to stand in the corner. If only he had been big and strong then he would not have taken such treatment lying down.

105

23.7.26. Midday.

T. : " Papa has known Uncle Julius for a very long time, hasn't he ? "

M. : " Yes, Uncle Julius is Papa's brother you know, they grew up together, like you and your brother."

T. : " Papa is allowed to kiss Uncle Julius, but you are not."

Discussion.—On a previous occasion we had mentioned that the children must not allow themselves to be kissed by strangers, and must not kiss them. T. now wants to state that F. may kiss Uncle Julius and prefaces his statement to this effect by a question about the degree of intimacy between the two. When a close relationship has been discovered, he approves of kissing ; but the sister-in-law is not allowed to do what the brother may.

106

25.7.26.   Afternoon.

J. : " I want to be a teacher." (*a*).

F. : " Why do you want to be a teacher ? "

J. : " I've learned something." (*b*).

F. : " Well, what have you learned ? "

J. : " Spheres and such squares, round spheres (*c*). Then I'll teach the children something, so that the children know everything, and when they are children (i.e. if they do what I shall do, and teach) they'll learn their children and at last the whole town has grown up and then every-body is dead (*d*). People grow on trees, don't they ? " (*e*).

F. : " Who told you that ? "

J. : " They grow near their mother's heart." (*f*).

T. : " Julius, I can read." (*g*).

J. : " Well, read then."

T. : (Takes a newspaper and looks into it.)

J. : " I can't hear anything."

T. : " Well, when Papa reads you can't hear anything either." (*h*).

F. : " What did you like best on the ferry, Julius ? " (*j*).

J. : " I liked the train best. How long it was ! One train and then another train, and then another and all the trains were hooked together. Then St's don't need to travel at all, they just walk through the train and they're at Doberan." (*k*).

F. : " But Uncle and Auntie St. don't want to go to Doberan, they want to go to Hamburg."

J. : " Then they can walk all through the train ; then all the trains are hooked together, dining-cars, cattle-trucks, passenger-coaches, and at last they've walked to Hamburg (*l*). They carry people who can't walk in stretchers. They have to lie quite still or else they are too heavy. They (i.e. the stretcher-bearers) must be strong, or else they can't carry them." (*m*).

F. : " Have you seen that ? "

J. : " Yes."

F. : " When did you see it ? "

J. : " I know it already." (*n*).

Discussion.—(*a*) A new hitherto unmentioned future profession, that of teacher, now appears. (*b*) J. wants to be a

teacher from the urge to impart knowledge. M. has shown
to the children coloured geometrical figures (*c*), used in a
lecture on child psychology.   These seem to J. sufficient
material to teach from.   (*d*) A whole series of generations
is to profit by his teaching activities, the one passing on
the knowledge gained to the next. Then his train of thought
proceeds rather by leaps than by stages : " the whole town
has grown up and everybody is dead."   It is only a step
from dying to being born.   (*e*) There may be here a faint
recollection of some story heard about people growing
on trees, but J. at once rejects this hypothesis when his
father questions him ; there occurs to him (*f*) what he has
previously heard about the beginning of human life. (*g*) The
conversation takes a new turn through T's half serious, half
joking statement that he can read. Against J's protest that
he can hear nothing T. skilfully advances the argument
that nothing is to be heard when even Papa reads (*h*).
(*j*) A new theme is here introduced by F.   The children
had been with their parents to the ferry coming from
Denmark, as we were to meet there some colleagues passing
through Rostock in the course of their journey. The children
had watched the shunting of the train in front of the ferry
with the most intense interest. So when F. asks about the
ferry, J. does not answer him, but begins to let his tongue
and his imagination run riot about the train. (*k*) The idea
that it is possible to reach one's destination by walking
through train after train coupled together, is a flight of
fancy which, as an adult can easily feel, would have a special
charm for a child.   J. has forgotten the real destination
of the St's, and so he mentions the first place that occurs
to him—Doberan.   When it is objected that Hamburg,
not Doberan is the destination, the new patent travelling
apparatus is turned in that direction, and the whole affair
is gone through again in detail.   The child's imagination
is still dependent on visual images, and so in making up his
train he uses all the kinds of railway rolling-stock known
to him. (*m*) On the way home from the ferry the children

had seen stretchers at a Red Cross depot. J. now speaks about those. He develops a theory of weight derived from his own experiences when carrying or being carried. The children are interested in ambulance work and workers because F. had often told them stories on this subject. (*n*) This does not mean that he has already seen it, but that he knows it from previous accounts he has heard.

107

28.7.26. Afternoon.

T. : (pointing to a Japanese tie-pin) " What's that ? "

F. : " That is a tie-pin."

T. : " So that people can see you come from Rostock ? " (*a*).

F. : " No, to keep the tie in place."

T. : " What is that on the tie-pin ? "

F. : " It is a Japanese landscape. Here is the mountain Fujiyama which is so high that it is always covered in snow even in Summer."

T. : " Then the people can go up and make snowballs and throw them into the town, and then people will say they are balls of cotton wool, but when they pick them up they'll find out that it's snow and then they'll say to others (in the street) ' Why are you throwing snowballs at us ? ' (Laughing) They won't know that people have thrown the snowballs from the mountain." (*b*).

Discussion.—The thought that a tie-pin could be used as a badge to denote which town a person belongs to is an extremely good original performance. We do not think that T. has ever heard anyone put forward or speak about such a possibility. (*b*) T. now imagines a new childish prank when he hears of snow-capped Fujiyama. How entertaining is the idea that the people in the town will not discover the source of the snowballs which they thought at first were balls of cotton wool, and that they will make the mistake of accusing passers-by of throwing snowballs. T. became really enthusiastic in imagining this scene.

108

1.8.26.   Morning at breakfast.

F. : " Theodor, when you think of Papa, what do you
do ? "

T. : " I hear you speak." (*a*).

F. : " What do I say ? "

T. : " When I am in bed at night you ask me how
I am." (*b*).

F. : " And what do you say then ? "

T. : " Very well." (*c*).

F. : " And what does Papa say ? "

T. : " Are you still thinking of nasty things ? Then I
say something else and I hope that I'll soon forget it." (*d*).

Discussion.—Our object was to determine whether T's
parents ever occurred in his world of ideas. We consider
it highly probable that from a certain age onwards, dialogue
becomes extremely significant, far above its enormous
immediate importance for social intercourse and social
influence. The new significance is due to the fact that the
child encounters in his mind, in certain situations, his parents
or other persons of his environment to whom he talks,
and that such conversations, taking place mentally, become
decisive factors in many things which the child either does
or leaves undone. If the child, thrown upon himself, learns
to resist impulsive tendencies, or to act in the spirit of his
educative influences, it is very probable the persons he
imagines to be present (either silent or speaking) who assist
him by their advice. When we speak of the voice of
conscience, there is probably behind the image (as so often
behind the figures of speech) a reality much more concrete
than the frequent use of the term in everyday life would
lead us to suspect. In the child, the voice of conscience is
the voice of those concerned in his education, and so primarily
that of the parents which the child hears mentally. In the
case of children with strongly developed visual power,
the warning, anxious face of father or mother may also
be present together with the voice. The more the process

of education is shared with others (as applies in the case of the child just starting school) and the more the warnings are freed from attachment to individual persons, with consequent substitution of more general principles for fixed rules of conduct in specific cases, the greater becomes the probability that the voice of conscience will lose its individual character and take on an impersonal form. Then, to some extent, the voice of public opinion is heard. We believe that our children were still in the first stage, and that it was chiefly us they heard when they were acting, not purely impulsively, but being warned or encouraged under the influence of former experiences. There are many indications of a development such as we have outlined above, and we should be unwilling to abandon it immediately as inaccurate, even if an insufficiency of childish self-observation should make its proof impossible. An essential condition for the correctness of our theory is of course that other people should in some way be mentally present to the child, even if they are not actually present. Few people will doubt that a five to six year old child can visualize human beings just as easily as inanimate objects, nor will any child psychologist dispute the existence of the representation (visualization) of objects in children. But without further proof we cannot admit that the child has mental intercourse with these visualized persons, whether it be carried on silently or in verbal conversation. We believe that the above conversation in all probability does furnish this proof. (*a*) Firstly, T. is not in the least surprised when F. asks him the first question, but at once he knows a suitable answer. " I hear you speak " implies a real experience which T. is referring to, for his description was not in any way suggested by the question. Taking into account the whole personality of the child, we consider it very improbable that he would have volunteered such information without a corresponding experience. We do not maintain that, during a mental meeting with F. a conversation did actually take place exactly as T. indicates in (*c*) and (*d*) when asked, but there may very well have been mental conversations of this same type. According to T's statements he occasionally suffered from being obliged to think when lying in bed of " nasty " things (by which he probably means disturbing things such as witches, etc.) and then it is very probable that on such occasions he takes refuge with his father, who on previous similar occasions has been able to console him. From mere reproduction of conversations which have really taken place we must make the further step to those in which, by referring to earlier experiences, a purely imaginary situation gives rise to a mental conversation. A particularly effective cause of the mental visualization of F. and M. must arise from former situations, whose material contained a conflict.

109

7.8.26.   Evening, after washing.   F. is away from home. T. comes from the place where he has been performing his toilet into the room where J. is.

T. :   " Papa has come back, Papa has come back."

J. :   " Where is he, where is Papa ? " (*a*).

T. :   (points to the kitchen) " Papa's there."

J. :   " Why doesn't Papa come in ?   Papa must come in." (*b*).

M. :   " Theodor is teasing you, you know Papa's away."

J. :   " Theodor, are you teasing me ? "

T. :   " Yes, I was teasing you."

J. :   " You rascal, now I'll tease you too.   I am (pause), I am a wolf " (J. growls aloud) (*c*).

T. :   (afraid) " You are Julius, aren't you ? "

J. :   " No, I am a wolf." (*d*).

T. :   (Becomes very frightened.)

M. :   " It is only Julius and only a joke."   (In order to appease, T., M. has to repeat this several times.)

Discussion.—The children like to tease each other in fun.   It is really curious how crudely they proceed in such cases, and yet always succeed in producing an effect.   (*a, b*) When T. calls out, J. is thoroughly convinced that F. has returned. An adult of course would not have succumbed to the suggestion, for under those circumstances M. would have behaved quite differently from what she did. But what appears scarcely credible is that the older T. is taken in by the crude deception of his younger brother, even after revenge has been expressly threatened and not even been postponed to some favourable situation where suggestion can play its part (as is done for instance on 1st April), but immediately put into execution. And what does J. do? He simply declares he is a wolf and growls as well as he can, in order to indicate a wolf (c). There is no change at all in his external appearance; for instance he has not previously gone out of the room and then come in again, so as to simulate a transformation. The very first attack makes T. frightened and he attempts to induce his brother to confess that he is really Julius. But J. insists that he is a wolf and then T. becomes more and more afraid. We must expressly emphasize that T. really *is* afraid and is by no means feigning fright in order to please J. T's terror is so great that M. has to intervene to reassure him. Once more we ask, along the line of questions raised in conversation 35: Does T. really believe that he is no longer dealing with his brother, but with a wolf? The situation is just the same as that of the mother changed into a bear. T. actually believes J. to be his brother and a wolf, all in one. We may also add here that probably T. is not alone in falling victim to the magical effect of the word, but that even the magician himself (i.e. even J.) is convinced that he is a wolf. It is just the same with the Shaman who by his own magic power has assumed animal form and thereby feels himself to be an animal. It is just as well that the children do not fully realize what power over other children this word-magic gives them, for otherwise they could misuse it to an alarming degree and keep other children subject to them through its power. Certainly no moral considerations would restrain them from such a misuse of this power.

Here we include four fragmentary conversations of an episodic nature. These minor events may serve to characterize the two children without our adding any further comments.

8.8.26. The two children are eating ice-cream. F. asks the children to give him some of theirs. T. complies with the request, but J. refuses.

F. : " Why won't you give me any, Julius ? "

J. : " Because I shall only have a bit for myself then."

9.8.26. The two children are eating ice-cream. F. takes a little from T's plate, without any objection being raised. Then F. takes some from J's plate.

J. : " You'll eat it all away from me."

9.8.26. On a picnic J. announces a physical necessity. He is held out, but at first without result. Only after some time is the desired result achieved.

J. : (Obviously to conceal his confusion) " I was teasing you."

T. : " Such affairs (!) aren't joked about."

9.8.26. Something had taken place on the beach. J. reports it with the words " I didn't see it, but I know it ". Here, therefore, the important distinction is made between knowledge gained through one's own perception and that based on other considerations.

10.8.26. Forenoon. T. and J. wanted to play bride and bridegroom. M. dresses up quite simply to suit the part, scatters flowers and then acts as the registrar.

M. : " What is your name, dear bride ? "

J. : " Miss Lieschen Katz." (a).

M. : " How old ? "

J. : " Five years." (b).

M. : " Where do you live ? "

J. : " Number six." (c).

M. : " Which town ? "

J. : " In Cassel." (d).

M. : " What street ? "

J. : " Mecklenburg Street." (e).

M. : " What is your profession, what do you work at ? "

J. : " I am a gardener." (f).

M. : " What is your name, my dear bridegroom ? "

T. : (archly) " I am called Ursula Schnickschnack." (g).

M. : " My dear bridegroom, are you called Mr. Ursula Schnickschnack ? "

J. : (interrupting) " Yes, that is my father's name." (h).

M. : " How old are you, my dear bridegroom ? "

T. : " I am twenty." (j).

M. : " Where did you live ? "

T. : " In Paul Street in France." (k).

M. : " What is your profession ? "

T. : " I am a railwayman." (l).

Discussion.—Scarcely a day passed about this time without some character play being acted. The present theme is a new departure, and it cannot be said with certainty how the children came across it. The improvisations (*a, b, c, d, e, f*) were invented quite skilfully by J., with the one exception of the statement of his own age. He thinks of Cassel because that town was often spoken about, as many relatives live there. He calls the street " Mecklenburg Street " in honour of his own home. The profession he mentions has never been suggested before. T. shows himself to be much more alive to the humour of the situation than J. (*g*) He gives a feminine name in order to make fun of the registrar, for of course he knows perfectly well that as bridegroom he ought to have a masculine Christian name. Both Christian and surname are witty inventions. (*h*) J., who has not been asked, takes it upon himself to answer the astonished question of the registrar. From his reply we see that he has by no means a correct impression of the relationship of bride and bridegroom. (*j*) The age given is within the bounds of possibility. (*k*) This street name does occur in Rostock, but it occurs to T. that it would have been better to have chosen a fictitious street name, and so, to heighten the illusion he moves it away from Rostock to France. (*l*) As his profession the bridegroom gives one of the previously mentioned future professions.

112

10.8.26. Afternoon.

M. : " Auntie O., do you know that T. got some new shoes to-day ? Or else he'd have lost his toes, which were already peeping out, and then we'd have had to get them again from the lost property office."

T. : " What is a lost property office ? "

M. : " When anything is found in the street, it must be handed over to the police."

T. : " Arms and legs are handed over to the lost property office too, aren't they ? " (a).

M. : " Why, what do you mean ? "

T. : " Well, when we go to the Institute, then we meet people who have lost their arms and legs, and the policeman has certainly had the arms and legs handed to him. (b).

Discussion.—(a, b) As F. had carried out researches on people who had lost a limb, they had occasionally been mentioned in the parent's conversation. Near to the Psychological Institute there was a Welfare Bureau for people who had lost limbs, so that T. had had an opportunity of seeing such people, and inquiring about them. By misconstruing the figure of speech, T. takes the loss of members literally. And so it must be possible to get them back again from the Lost Property Office. If only it were !

113

11.8.26. Morning. M. and T. are visiting a family and see a baby drinking from the bottle. T. looks on for a time and then says " You are the best Mama in the whole world for letting me drink from you ". (a).

11.8.26. Afternoon.

T. : " Mama, I love you so much because you bore me (gave me birth)." (b).

Discussion.—We include these two short statements of T. because they appear to us eminently suitable for demonstrating what a beautiful bond of love can be forged between mother and child by an explanation adapted to the child's age, instead of the fairy tale about the stork. (a) T. did not know that the mother's breast is better for children than the bottle, and so he is only thinking of the intimate relationship which has existed between his mother and himself through her offering her breast, and he is thankful to M. for this. (*b*) Here too the feeling of gratitude is expressed to his mother for bearing him and giving him life.

114

15.8.26. T. and J. are playing at shop with Elli.

E. : " I should like some dyes please."
J. : " We have only these dyes."
E. : " Here is your money, is it right ? "
J. : " Yes."
E. : " What is your name ? "
J. : " I am called Ludwig and he is called Peter." (*a*).
T. : " No, that's not my name, I'm called Wilhelm." (*b*).
E. : " Where do you live ? "
T. : " In Saxony, Berlin Street."
E. : " What number ? "
T. : " Number nine."
J. : " Elli, write a letter."
E. : " To whom ? "
J. : " To Punch." (*c*).
E. : " Where does Punch live ? "
J. : " In Friedrich Franz Street, with a cobbler." (*d*).
E. : " I'll write to Punch."

Discussion.—(*a*) J. gives names which occur only rarely even in his circle of acquaintances. (*b*) T. immediately protests against the name given to him, and mentions his own second Christian name. (*c, d*) It is not easy to say what causes J. to think of Punch in this connection. The street J. mentions does exist in Rostock. The choice of a cobbler as landlord for Punch is emotionally extremely good.

115

15.8.26. Afternoon. M. is walking along the street with the children.

M. : (sees a caterpillar) " Let's take this caterpillar home with us and look closely at it." (M. wraps the caterpillar in a leaf.)

J. : " Yes, let's take this wild cat (!) home, lock it in a box and put bars in front so that it can't break out." (a).

T. : " Oh Mama, how brave you are." (b).

Discussion.—The fact that J., under the influence of sound association, turns the caterpillar into a wild cat is not so very surprising, but it is quite unexpected that T., under the suggestive influence of J's remarks, should also take the caterpillar for a dangerous animal and praise his mother for her bravery. (b)   His praise is meant seriously, not intended as a joke.

116

16.8.26.   Evening in bed.

J. : " Mama, I've never been in the country, can't we go now ? " (a).

M. : " Now ?   There aren't any trains at night."

J. : " But there are those trains you can sleep in. Grandmama came at night to Wustrow." (b).

M. : " Well, what shall we do then ? "

J. : " Let's pack the trunks, dress ourselves and set off. Give me the bell." (c).

M. : " Which bell ? "

J. : " The one I've made for Papa." (d).

T. : " Mama, is Uncle K. grown up ? " (e).

M. : " Yes."

T. : " But you're not, are you ? "

M. : " Why not ? "

T. : " Well you've still got a mama, haven't you ? " (f).

M. : " But one can still have a mama, even if one *is* grown up."

T. : " When did Papa's parents die ? " (g).

M. : " That was a long time ago."

Discussion.—(a) Of course J. has already been often " to the country " and even now he is at Warnemünde, but up till now he has not brought the content of the term " in the country " into line with his own experience. That is what is expressed in his statement. (b) J. has already heard of sleeping cars. How fine it would be just to ride in a train in which one can sleep ! (c) J. would certainly never hesitate for a moment about setting out on the spur of the moment at midnight. He is to take with him on his journey the bell which he has made for his absent father (d). Even though, as a child psychologist, one is prepared for most things, yet one is at times surprised by totally unexpected questions. For instance it has happened that J. has asked in broad daylight " Is it evening now ? " when the question should have been impossible for obvious reasons. In such cases it is discovered that quite immaterial circumstances may appear to the child as extremely important, as for instance in this latter case, the serving of a dish which usually is only eaten in the evening. How can T. ask if Uncle K. is grown up when he can obviously convince himself of the true state of affairs with his own eyes ? But he really means something else. What he means is, whether Dr. K's parents are still alive. For T. it is an essential part of being grown up, that one should no longer have any parents (probably in the sense : no longer *need* any) and so he thinks M. cannot be grown up because she still has a mama (f). (g) The question about F's parents, of whose death he has heard, makes it clear that he considers his father as grown up.

117

18.8.26. G. is telling about a children's party at which Uncle H. was present.

J. : " The boys were separated from the girls."

G. : " Yes, you know that."

J. : " Because boys are rough and girls gentle." (a).

G. : " Yes."

J. : " But Heidi B. is rough too, because she grew up rough." (b).

G. : " Uncle H. lost his belt at the party."

J. : " You can't go about without a belt, it looks so slovenly. In O. (where the party took place) it is as hot as where the negroes live." (c).

N

T. : " No, it's not as hot there as it is where the negroes live." (*d*).

J. : " Be quiet and let Grandma tell the story."

Discussion.—(*a*) An explanation for the segregation of the sexes which is discovered independently by J.   Then it occurs to him immediately, that Heidi B. (conv. 14) is an exception to the general rule that girls are gentle and reserved ; that is of course an honour for the little friend. (*c*) A calm acceptance of this beltless situation is not possible for J., he must express his reproaches to Uncle H.   The degree of heat in O. is emotionally exaggerated, so that T. has to recall his brother to reality (*d*).   (*e*) J. condemns his brother to silence : now he wants to hear further accounts from G.

118

19.8.26.   The children have just got new sailor suits which they are putting on.

M. : " When Papa comes back from his journey, dress yourselves as sailors, and go to the station and then Papa won't recognize you."

J. : " Is Papa coming to-day ? "

M. : " No, he'll be away a few days yet.   Then we'll go to the station and Papa will say ' These sailors look very like my little boys ', and he'll ask ' What are your names ? ' "

T. : " I'll say ' Wilhelm Theodor Katz '." (*a*).

M. : " Then Papa will say ' Oh, so then you're my little boy '."

T. : " Yes, that's much nicer, too." (*b*).

M. : " And then Papa will give you the presents.   And Julius, what will you say ? "

J. : " I'll say my name is Wilhelm." (*c*).

M. : " Then Papa will go away."

T. : " And you won't get any presents." (*d*).

J. : " But the presents won't be unpacked at the station, they'll be given out later, at home.   I'll come home with you, Mama will change my clothes and then Papa will say, why there you are, and then he won't know that I was a sailor."(*e*).

M. : " And then you'll have played a trick on Papa ? "

J. : " Yes."

Discussion.—(*a*) T. does not want to have any share in playing a trick on F. at the station when he returns, probably because he fears that F. may be hurt if he does not see his boys at once ; this is shown by (*b*). In any case there is no egoistical motive here, for the presents F. has brought are only worked into the conversation later by M. And so he finds it quite in order that J., who does not want to reveal his identity to F., should lose his presents (*d*). The fact that J. will pretend to be Wilhelm does not mean that he is assuming his brother's person, but the name of a sailor, as is shown by (*e*). Very skilfully J. counters the threat that he will have to go without presents by pointing out that the presents will only be unpacked at home, and not immediately at the station. A quick change of clothes will transform him once more into J. and Papa will not suspect in the least that he was identical with the sailor. But the fact that nevertheless he will have played a trick on F. gives him enormous pleasure.

119

23.8.26. Afternoon on the beach. T. is talking to Heinz, a boy from the Kindergarten.

T. : (to Heinz, who is eating a cake) " Oh I should like to have a cake like that."

H. : " My father is a baker, we have plenty of cakes. There are many bakers in the town."

T. : " My father isn't a baker, he's a professor."

Discussion.—The sense probably requires the addition of an " only " before " a professor " ; we believe that T. would have preferred F. to be a baker and then he too could have cake every day.

120

23.8.26. T. and J. are undressing to go to bed and are as they do so playing that they are taking up quarters in a hotel.

J. : " Can't you undress yourself ? "

T. : (whom G. is helping to undress) " This is my maid, she helps me." (*a*).

J. : " Where is your little son ? Is he married yet ? " (b).

T. : " Yes." (The children get into bed.)

J. : " Where is your father ? "

T. : " He has gone away." (c).

J. : " I saw him, he sailed past me in a ship." (d).

T. : " Let's go to sleep now." (Closes his eyes.) (e).

J. : " Now let's get up." (f).

T. : " Let's wash ourselves."

J. : " Can you pour out some water for me ? "

T. : " Here is the soap. Mama, you see we're playing at washing our hands." (g). (J. knocks something over.) " Is anything broken ? "

J. : " No, or I should have to pay for it and I've no money. I gave the porter all my money." (h). (The children lie down in bed.) " Stick, stick to the wall, come you must go in Grandma's hand." (j).

Discussion.—One could speak here of a purpose game (Zweckspiel), since the undressing and evening toilet have been turned into a game. (a) As usually happens, adults present are included in the game, and here G. is raised to the dignity of a chambermaid. (b) Here the suitable tone of voice must be imagined, in which the inquiry about the little son is couched. (c) It is true that Father has gone away, but J. keeps to the game and maintains that he has seen him on a ship. (e) The children are now in bed and pretend to be asleep for a short time, then they get up again (f) and wash themselves properly (g). (h) There is a very noticeable anxiety in J's reply that he has no more money, as he has already given everything to the porter. (j) After getting into bed, J. occupies himself as a poet. Of late J. had tried more and more frequently to make rhymes, obviously stimulated by the little verses occurring in stories. This tendency, which has persisted and developed up to the present time has never been noticed in T. About the same time as the foregoing conversation for instance, he composed the rhyme : Kleckerman, put your old trousers on.[1]

[1] Studies of children as poets are given by A. Dyroff ; *Ueber das Seelenleben des Kindes*, 2nd ed., 1911.

121

25.8.26. Afternoon.

M. : " Theodor, you must go out."

T. : " Why can't I stay in with you ? "

M. : " If children get plenty of fresh air they grow up strong and healthy.

T. : " Oh, so Uncle P. probably didn't go out very much because he only grew a little, or perhaps he was too rough."

Discussion.—Uncle P. is a somewhat deformed acquaintance, but we had never drawn T's attention to his small stature. T. now thinks that by utilizing what he has just heard he can explain why Uncle P. has remained so small : probably he did not go out enough into the fresh air. However a second hypothesis is immediately added : perhaps this Uncle remained so small because he was too rough.

122

27.9.26. Evening.

T. : " Grandma, when the giant Goliath lay in his grave his legs would stick out, wouldn't they ? " (*a*).

G. : " No, his legs didn't stick out."

T. : " Where was the giant born ? " (*b*).

G. : " I don't know."

T. : " Mama's sure to know." (*c*).

J. : " The giant was born in Giant Town." (*d*).

G. : " Yes, there is a Giant Town where giants are born."

Discussion.—(*a*) After a long interval the giant Goliath is brought on the carpet again. Only a child would be anxious as to whether his legs stuck out of the grave. T. asks the question about the burial of Goliath quite spontaneously, for it had never been spoken of by anyone else. (*b*) The question is probably to be understood as : Where is the town or the place in which such giants (not only Goliath) are born ? (*c*) shows what confidence T. has in his mother's knowledge. (*d*) An ingenious solution of the problem raised. What is tautology for an adult is a completely satisfying explanation for the child.

16.9.26. Evening.

J. : " Mama, may I sleep in your bed ? " (a).

M. : " No, children may not sleep with grown-ups ; it makes both children and grown-ups ill."

J. : " But I do so want to sleep with you." (b).

M. : " I have been speaking to a doctor, and he told me that one shouldn't sleep with children."

T. : " If a doctor says that, then it is so ; a doctor knows everything." (c).

M. : " Shall we pray."

T. : " No, praying is dull." (d)

J. : (clasps his hands). " I will be good, I will be good, I will be good, I will not do anything naughty."

M. : " Amen."

J. : " What does Amen mean ? "

M. : " Amen means ' so be it '. Theodor, have you done anything wrong to-day ? "

T. : " I don't think so. If I had done anything naughty then I should think of it at once, it would occur to me straight away." (e).

J. : " Ask me." (f).

M. : " Julius, have you done anything wrong ? "

J. : " I played at trains to-day and climbed on the hill." (g).

M. : " Was it wrong to play at trains and climb on the hill ? "

J. : " Grandma was afraid." (h).

M. : " If Grandma is afraid, you must not climb on the hill."

J. : " You must write a note to Grandma, to tell her not to be afraid." (j).

T. : (completing) " When Julius climbs on the hill."

J. : " You know, Theodor, I was playing at trains and I was so afraid when Grandma cried out ; I really thought the policeman was coming." (k).

T. : " Did Grandma catch you ? " (l).

J. : " No, Grandma didn't catch me." (m).

Discussion. (a) The children slept in their own room, each in his own bed. Often they used to come in early in the morning, and were then allowed to slip into bed with their parents for a short time. To break them of this habit, M. now brings forward the medical authority in opposition to J's request. (*b*) Whereas J. overrides this authority by pointing out the greatness of his desire, his elder brother bows to it. What boundless confidence in doctors T. reveals by (*c*). (*d*) The unexpected refusal to pray is explained by the child's unusual tiredness on this evening. Probably nothing of any consequence had happened which ought to have been confessed. (*e*) T. characterizes the psychological position quite correctly. (*f*) As yet J. has not got so far as to begin the confessions spontaneously, but as compared with formerly he has made an advance, for now he really has something to confess, even if what he brings forward (*g*) does not at first look very like a confession. By his reckless climbing he had caused his Grandmother to be afraid (*h*) and now he feels this as an oppressive guilt. (*j*) J. thinks that if it is given to Grandmother in writing she will no longer need to be afraid and that will have a good effect. (*k*) In her anxiety about J's safety, G. must have threatened him with the policeman, and this in its turn made J. afraid. (*l, m*) T's rather roguish question is denied by J. with pride and satisfaction.

124

19.9.26. F. is using the typewriter, T. is lying on the sofa and listening to the noise of the machine.

T. : " Do you know, Papa, when you use the typewriter I say to you : perlicke, perlacke."

Discussion.—The words perlicke, perlacke make up the magic formula or spell used in many fairy tales. Such a fairy tale had been recently told to the children. The rhythmically-tapping noise of the typewriter working recalls the words to T's consciousness. It must be admitted that T. achieves a good performance in connecting the tapping of the typewriter onomatopœically with the magic spell. It is not a question of the formation of a new word, but nevertheless of a most suitable application of an existing word-formation to represent a series of acoustic impressions. The reproduction of the words perlicke, perlacke takes place by association because of the similarity in sound ; but the child performs a creative action in that he does not accept this similarity passively, but rather lifts it out of its sensory neutrality, and utilizes it descriptively in his statement to F. Neither this utterance nor any of the numerous others in our conversations is to be explained without assuming willing to be an elementary function, directed to the production of utterances.[1]

125

19.9.26. Evening in bed.

T. : " Mama, there's still something we must do." (a).

M. : " Pray ? "

T. : " Yes." (clasps his hands and says very softly) " I will be good, I will not do anything naughty."

J. : " I will pray with you too." (Prays.)

M. : " Theodor, have you anything to say to me ? "

T. : " I don't know of anything. Perhaps you can help me ? " (b).

M. : " Theodor, were you good to-day with Auntie O. in the street, with Grandma, with Elli ? "

T. : " I wasn't at home all day."

M. : " Were you good in Warnemünde ? "

T. : " Yes."

M. : " Now I'll go to Julius."

J. : " Let me pray, I'll start, go." (c).

M. : " Start now."

J. : " I will be good, I will not do anything naughty. Now ask me."

M. : " Have you anything to tell me ? "

J. : " I'll think about it again. Yes, I took a ribbon from Theodor." (d).

M. : " Did the ribbon belong to you ? "

J. : " No, it belonged to Theodor." (e).

[1] Lindworsky in his experimental work has been the chief exponent of willing as a specific process.   It is also noteworthy that G. E. Müller at the Leipzig Congress for Experimental Psychology propounded, for cases of arbitrary movement, an impulse theory in place of the theory of the attention of the will. (*Congress Report*, Jena, 1924.)

T. : " Yes, it was my ribbon."

M. : " Why did you take the ribbon from Theodor ? "

J. : " Because I wanted to have a ribbon." (*f*).

M. : " But one of yours was lying on the table."

J. : " No, I had no ribbon, so Mama took me with her and gave me a ribbon."

T. : " Why did you want such a long ribbon ? "

J. : " Yes, I wanted such a long ribbon." (*g*).

M. : " Julius, did you do anything good to-day ? "

J. : " Yes, everything else was good. Mama, if a house is on fire, that's worse, isn't it, than if a child is on fire ? " (*h*).

M. : " If a child is on fire it is very serious."

J. : " Yes, but if a whole house is on fire it's worse." (*k*).

M. : " An empty house ? "

J. : " A full house."

M. : " That would scarcely happen, for the people run out as soon as fire breaks out."

J. : " Yes, but everyone doesn't notice it at once."

M. : " Oh, but someone notices it and tells the others.

J. : " Then they send for the fire brigade. Is the fire brigade always up ? " (*l*).

M. : " Someone keeps watch day and night at the fire-station."

J. : " What does watch mean ? " (*m*).

M. : " A man who is always on the look out."

J. : " Then they tell him " (that a fire has broken out).

M. : " Then the fire brigade comes on a motor."

J. : " The fire brigade doesn't ride on a motor, does it ? " (*n*).

M. : " Yes, the fire brigade rides on a big motor."

J. : " Then the fire brigade puts out the fire."

M. : " The fire brigade has big ladders, which are placed to the windows and they carry the children down."

J. : " And down below the firemen stand with big sheets, and at the top they give you a push and down you fly into the sheet. It's very hard to be a fireman." (*o*).

M. : " Would you like to be a fireman ? "

J. : " No, I wanted to be a poet (!), but now I should like to be a captain again." (*p*).

M. : " How does one become a poet ? "

J. : " You learn how." (*q*).

T. : " That can't be learned." (*r*).

M.: " How will you learn ? "

J.: " You build yourself a house, go into it and write a book." (*s*).

M.: " What kind of book would you like to write ? "

J.: " Like Berni." (*t*).

T.: " But you want to be a sea-captain, don't you ? "

J.: " I did want to be a captain, but you have to be able to swim, and I shouldn't like to do that." (*u*).

T.: " But you can swim already." (*v*).

J.: " No, not yet."

T.: " Yes, you can swim properly."

M.: " Now good night. I'll go and see what Papa is doing."

J.: " Hit Papa." (*w*).

T.: " No, don't. It's so dreadful, you shouldn't even say it." (*x*).

J.: "But Auntie O. hits me even when I'm good, so that I go all red and blue and green, then you could paint from me. You only need to take a paint brush and place a piece of paper beside me and you can paint from me." (*y*).

Discussion.—(*a*) About this time it has become a necessity for T. to pray at night ; if it is forgotten, he reminds us of it. (*b*) He himself cannot remember any naughty action, but he asks M. to help him in searching his conscience. It appears, however, that he really has done nothing naughty. (*c*) J. has indeed prayed already with T., but now wants to do so again, on his own. The " go " is much more suitable for the start of a sporting event than for the beginning of a prayer. (*d, e, f, g*) After some thought, J. remembers the sin he has committed. The reason given for the theft is characteristic of J. and probably of all children at this age. It suffices to *want* something belonging to another person in order to believe that one has a lawful claim to that thing. (*h*) The conversation takes a completely new turn. J. has as yet no idea that the value of human life cannot be compared to that of other goods. (*k*) He probably wishes to state in his comparison, that if a house is on fire, the flames are larger than when a child is burning, and quantitatively that is worse. At (*l*), J. brings up his beloved fire brigade.

One might almost say, that just as the incendiary sets fire to a house for the pleasure of watching the firemen at work, so J. sets a house on fire in his imagination in order to enjoy the imaginative description of all that takes place then. (*m*) J. has up to now never met the word watch in connection with the fire brigade, and he immediately inquires its meaning. (*n*) J. is thinking of the ordinary cars in the street, and so he questions whether the firemen will use such a vehicle ; to the child the essential is not the method of movement, but the external form of the vehicle, and this is of course different from others in the case of the fire brigade. (*o*) Notice the naïve description of rescue by means of the sheet. But however much he takes delight in the fire brigade, he himself does not want to be a fireman ; he does not give a reason for his refusal. (*p*) It is unusual for a four-year-old child to make even a temporary choice of the profession of poet—a choice which he soon rejects. (*q, s, t*) Here we learn how to become a poet. T's interjection, that one cannot learn to be a poet (*r*) reveals his sensitive appreciation of the situation. (*u*) The profession of sea-captain has here been temporarily renounced, because one would have to be able to swim. J. seems to think that a captain must be constantly swimming. (*v*) To our great surprise J. did really learn to swim a little without any help from us, during his daily bathes at Warnemünde. (*w*) This utterance springs from pure exuberance, for there was not the slightest cause for any aggressive feelings towards F. (*x*) T. takes J's request seriously and will not be a party to any ill-treatment of F. " You shouldn't even say it." (*y*) A strange performance of the childish imagination, in which J's natural roguishness takes control of the associatively developed chains of ideas, or more correctly, allows itself to be directed by them.

126

21.9.26. Evening in bed. T. is doing gymnastics.
T. : " Mama, this is how we did at Auntie M's. Yes, just like this."

M. : " Would you like to do gymnastics again at Auntie M's ? "

J. : " Yes, I should like to."

T. : " I'd rather dig a hole in the sand at Warnemünde." (*a*).

J. : " I've made a mistake. I don't want to do gymnastics either, it makes you so tired when you come home. I'd prefer to dig a water-hole too. Then you can play ice-cream seller with the mud." (*b*).

T. : " Pooh ! "

J. : " Yes, you make mud and then ask ' do you want some ice-cream ? ' and then you pretend to eat." (*c*).

T. : " But you know you can't eat mud." (*d*).

J. : " No, you only pretend to." (*e*).

T. : " Wet sand is clay, isn't it ? " (*f*).

M. : " No, wet sand is not clay. When you go for a walk and see a bricklayer at work, ask him to show you some clay."

T. : " I should like to bring some home, wrapped in paper."

J. : " Yes, and bring some stones with you too, then we can build a house. We'll look for glass and a frame in the street, and then we'll put a window in." (*g*).

T. : " No, you are silly, silly." (*h*).

M. : " No, Julius is not silly, he is only small ; you must tell him where to get frames from."

T. : " He ought to know that frames are not found in the street." (*j*).

M. : " Where do we get frames from ? "

T. : " From the window-cleaner." (*k*).

M. : " From the window-cleaner ? "

T. : " From the joiner." (*l*).

M. : " Yes, from the joiner—and the glass ? "

J. : " From Mr. Glass." (*m*).

T. : " From Albert M., he's a glazier." (*n*).

J. : " Yes, from the glazier."

M. : " Have you been to a glazier's ? "

T. : " Yes, with Auntie O. Mama, how old will you be ? " (*o*).

M. : " I don't know."

T. : " But you'll have this birthday and next, certainly." (*p*).

Discussion.—The children had taken part in children's gymnastics at Warnemünde for several weeks. Although T. especially had been extremely delighted, yet he now prefers to dig a water-hole (*a*). Then J. reconsiders and decides also that a water-hole with its facilities for play is really more interesting (*b*, *c*). The first reason stated, that gymnastics makes him tired is only a pretext. (*d*) When T. raises the objection that the mud can't be eaten, J. stresses the fact that he only means it in play (*e*). (*f*) The assumption that wet sand is clay is a good mistake, for things can be shaped from wet sand, just as from clay. T. on one occasion watched a lady of our acquaintance modelling M. in clay, and from that time he repeatedly expressed the desire to shape things in clay, just as Robinson Crusoe did. (*g*) J. develops now a complete programme for building a house. T. is outraged at J's naïve assumption that complete window frames for house construction may be found in the street (*h*, *j*). At first he himself gives a false source for the supply of window frames (*k*), but then corrects himself (*l*). (*m*) It is a thoroughly childish idea that glass may be obtained from a Mr. Glass. T. gives the correct source (*n*). At (*o*), the conversation takes a new turn. The question does not mean " how old will you be on your next birthday ? " but " how long will you live ? " The assurance that M. will certainly celebrate this birthday and the next is meant to express that T. wishes his mother a very long life. For a child, two birthdays means an extremely long time.

127

22.9.26. Evening in bed.

T. : " Mama, are there still spots on my neck ? " (From a bandage fixed with adhesive plaster.)

M. : " Yes, a few, I'll rub them off for you to-morrow."

T. : " They are still sticking, but they'll be gone by my wedding, won't they ? " (*a*).

M. : " When are you going to get married ? "

T. : " In four, five, or seven years." (*b*).

M. : " How old will you be in seven years ? "

T. : " I don't know."

M. : " How much is five and seven ? "

T. : " I don't know."

M. : " It's twelve, and then you'll be about as old as W. G., you'll still be at school then. Thirty is the time for marrying."

T. : " Then I'll get married when I'm thirty." (c).

M. : " Where will you live then ? "

T. : " In Italy."

M. : " Why in Italy ? "

T. : " Because there are pears and apricots there." (d).

J. : " I should like to live in the country ; you can pick everything for yourself there, and there's roast meat, hm, hm ! " (e).

T. : " You are always saying hm, hm."

J. : " Mama, in the country you can pick everything for yourself and there is roast meat." (f).

T. : " Mama, why are the countries smaller than the towns ? " (g).

M. : " Do you mean the villages ? "

T. : " Yes, the villages."

M. : " The towns have spread because there are a great many people there."

T. : " Mama, is it nicer to live in the country ? "

M. : " What do you say to that, Julius ? "

J. : " I should prefer to live in the country, and when I get married I'll live in the country." (h).

T. : " You'll live in Berlin or in some other town, but not in the country."

M. : " You'll see later on."

T. : " Mama, why had the woman no parrots to sell ? " (We had bought a salamander for the children from an animal dealer.) (j).

M. : " I expect she had none."

T. : " Mama, will you buy me some goldfish to-morrow ? "

M. : " No, Theodor, we bought a salamander to-day, so we can't buy something else to-morrow."

T. : " But the day after to-morrow, or next week ? "

M. : " Yes, some-time we'll buy you some goldfish."

T. : " How many salamanders had the woman ? " (k).

M. : " I think she had four."

J. : " Mama, come and sit by me."

T. : " If I don't go to sleep come back to me."

M. : " I think you'll soon go to sleep, Theodor. It will be better if we say good night to each other at once."

T. : " Good night."

J. : " Come, Mama, sit nearer to me."

M. : " Yes, I am already quite close to you."

J. : " Mama, how many salamanders had the woman ? " (*l*).

M. : " I think she had four."

J. : " How did you know ? "

M. : " I looked into the salamander house."

J. : " But if the woman is selfish and won't sell us any, then we'll have to break the glass and get in through the window." (*m*).

M. : " No, you may not get in through the window, and you may not break the glass."

J. : " But if the woman is selfish, and if she allows us to get in through the window ? " (*n*).

M. : " She won't allow that. Those who want to go into the shop must go through the door."

J. : " We could climb into the chimney, and get in through the fire-place." (*o*).

M. : " Then you'd be as black as a salamander, the painters would only need to paint a red stripe on you."

J. : " That would be fine." (*p*).

Discussion.—(*a*) The mention of the wedding is quite serious ; we see both here and in statement (*b*) that T. still has quite indefinite ideas about all relationships time. (*c*) Nor of course does T. understand what is meant by a space of thirty years, but he subjects himself to M's standard. (*d*) The choice of his future place of residence and the reasons given for this choice are just as characteristic of T. as is the totally different choice of J. (*e, f*). T. has very little patience with the stress J. lays on the culinary side of the business. At (*g*), the conversation takes another turn, but then comes back again to the previous question of residence (*h*). The great event of the day had been the purchase of a salamander. From the salamander, a strange and new creature to the children, it is an obvious step to

the equally strange parrot (*j*). Even though all the salamanders cannot be acquired, it is of importance to discover
how many there were there altogether (*k*). J. too returns
to this question in the conversation he carries on with
M.(*l*). J. has as yet no proper idea of the commercial transac-
tion of selling (*m*) ; he thinks selling is akin to presenting—
perhaps because his parents present what they have bought
to him—and so he thinks it possible that the woman did
not want to sell because of selfishness. To meet this situation
he at once propounds plans for deeds of violence. (*n*) When
objections are raised he persists in his opinion, but considers
that possibly the woman would raise no objection to an
entrance through the window. He does not observe the inner
contradiction in the statement. Then the adventurous
spirit suggests a quite different way into the shop to him (*o*)
and he readily appreciates the description painted by
M. (*p*).

128

23.9.26. Evening in bed. At first the children are
playing with tram tickets.

J. : " For my child too (a ticket). This is my child, a
little girl ; she goes to the kindergarten."

T. : (turning to M) " How old are you ? "

M. : " Four and a half."

T. : " Four and a half, yes, that's all right."

J. : (pointing to F.) " Let the little boy come too."

T. : (asks F.) " How old are you ? " (F. pretends to be
dumb. The children laugh, but after a time T. becomes
uneasy and calls out anxiously " Papa ". F. pulls his coat
over his head, and the children laugh heartily. When F.
begins to walk away J. calls after him " Papa, be funny
again ".)

M. : " Theodor, have you anything to tell me ? "

T. : " We haven't prayed yet." (*a*).

M. : " Then let us pray."

T. : (quite softly) " I will be good . . . Amen."

J. : " Mama, you always stay such a long time with T.
and such a short time with me." (*b*).

M. : " Theodor will fall asleep in a moment and then I'll come to you."

T. : " Mama, I'll warm your hand for you."

J. : " It takes too long."

M. : " I'll go to J. and quieten him, so that he won't disturb your sleep."

T. : " Yes."

M. : " Good night, sleep well."

T. : " Good night, Mama."

M. : " Julius, do you want to tell me anything ? "

J. : " To-day I trod on Auntie O's foot." (c).

M. : " What do you say when you tread on anyone's foot ? "

J. : " I don't know."

M. : " You say ' I'm sorry, I beg your pardon '."

J. : " I took the little girl of Auntie O's sister by the hand." (d).

M. : " Is that good or naughty ? "

J. : " Good. I wanted to play with her horse too, but she began to scream and I thought she'd fall on her nose. (e). (J. holds a thin sheet of paper against the light and shouts :) " Look Mama, I can see my hand through the ticket too." (G. comes.) " Grandma, you can see your hand through the tram ticket ! " (f).

Discussion.—The first part of the conversation is a typical character-play, in which the adults present are included. The conversation gets its experimental character by F. pretending to be dumb. We were very anxious to discover how the children would react to dumbness. It is very illuminating that J. was extremely amused at it, whereas T. became very uneasy. He tried to make F. speak properly again. The second part of the conversation is introduced by M. with the words " have you anything to tell me ? " We no longer use the form "have you done anything naughty" in the evening confessions in order to avoid suggesting to the child that he must always have done something naughty. (a) The evening prayer has already become a necessity to T., so that he himself reminds us of praying. (b) J. feels, though quite wrongly, that he is taking second place to T. The motive

o

is once again the feeling that the rights of the younger child are being infringed upon. (c) J. has learned to confess, and already tells quite spontaneously even his slightest misdemeanours when the evening " searching of conscience " takes place. (d) As compensation for his misdeed J. now reports a good action. As we see from (e) he considers the little girl as deficient ; she is too sensitive when played with as one does with a boy. (f) While playing with the tram ticket J. has accidentally discovered that his hand can be seen through the paper when both are in the correct position in relation to the light. He reports his discovery proudly to his grandmother also.

129

28.9.26.   Evening in bed.

T. : " Mama, what are you giving Papa for his birthday ? " (1st October.)

M. : " I haven't thought about that yet."

T. : " Aren't you ashamed of yourself ? " (a).

M. : " But there's still time to get something to-morrow."

J. : " A block of chocolate ? " (b).

M. : " And a cake is coming."

T. : " Have you a cake already ? "

M. : " Yes."

T. : " But Papa has seen that already." (c).

M. : " Then I'll give Papa a box of sweets."

T. : " And then I'll get some of them, and Julius too if he'll be good." (d).

M. : " Julius really was good this afternoon."

J. : " Mama, let us pray, but only a bit." (e). (J. is very sleepy. He prays softly, but he is heard to repeat often " I will not do anything naughty ".)

M. : " I think you couldn't have prayed yesterday seeing that to-day was such a bad day ? "

J. : " No. I didn't pray yesterday." (f).

Discussion.—It is not surprising that F's approaching birthday forms the main topic of conversation. (a) T. is quite indignant that M. has not yet thought about the presents F. is to receive, whilst he himself has been busy for days on little things he is making. (*b*) Of course the children ascribe to F. desires similar to their own, and so chocolate is mentioned as a present before anything else. (*c*) A birthday present that has already been seen is no longer a surprise and so is not a real birthday present at all. (*d*) Of course they are counting on some crumbs from the birthday table falling into their little mouths. J. had been very disobedient in the morning ; for instance he had refused to come for a walk with us. And now the terrible fear is awakened in him, that perhaps he will get less consideration on the great birthday, and so he takes refuge in prayer (*e*). It must be brief because he is tired, but it is touching to hear how in order to get strength he continually repeats " I will not do anything naughty ". J. appears already to have discovered that a firm good resolution is a great help, and even though answer (*f*) is suggested by M., yet it is along the lines of his own experience.

130

29.9.26. Morning in bed. J. wanted to come into M's bed, but he is not allowed, and T. also tries to prevent him.

T. : " If you aren't good you won't get anything from Papa's birthday table."

J. : " I'm not inquisitive (neugierig)."

T. : (laughing) " You don't mean inquisitive."

F. : " What is it then ? "

T. : " It's greedy (begierig), inquisitive (neugierig) is something else." (*a*).

F. : " Well, what is inquisitive ? "

T. : " You are being inquisitive now (i.e. you would like to know what you will get for your birthday.)." (*b*).

F. : " Yes, you are right. Julius must be good, or else he really won't get anything from the presents."

J. : " Then I'll get a big stick and hit you." (*c*).

F. : " Then we won't let you in."

J. : " Then I'll break the door down." (*d*).

F. : " And then we'll send for the police."

J. : " And then I'll fight the police." (*e*).

Discussion.—(*a*) That T. is able to make a clear distinction between the two similar sounding words "neugierig" and "begierig" must be counted as a good performance. His explanation of neugierig (inquisitive) by a reference to his father's state is also a skilful way of avoiding giving an explanation of the term in words (*b*). (*c, d, e*) J's three statements here characterize most aptly his resoluteness, and his intention of getting his own way, by force if need be. His defiance is fanned higher and higher.[1] J. is of an active disposition. His father's threats, however, have brought him almost to the verge of tears.

131

29.9.26. Morning. The children are returning from a visit to the pigeon which we were keeping at the institute for experimental purposes. They used to bring food for it daily at this time.

T. : " The poor pigeon is so lonely." (*a*).

M. : " Let's buy another pigeon ; a cock, then there will be a Mama and a Papa and they can have children."

T. : " Must there be a Papa and a Mama for children to come ? " (*b*).

M. : " There must always be a Papa and a Mama, and it's just the same with us too."

T. : " But Uncle P. won't have any children, there's no Mama there." (*c*).

M. : " No, Uncle P. has no wife and so he won't have any children."

J. : " But Uncle K. (demonstrator in the Institute) will have some children won't he ? " (*d*).

T. : " No, Uncle K. won't have any children either." (*e*).

J. : " Oh yes, Uncle K. will have some children. Won't he, Mama, won't Uncle K. have some children ? " (*f*).

M. : " No, Uncle K. has no wife and so he won't have any children either."

Discussion.—(*a*) We had occasionally mentioned that the pigeon might feel lonely, and T. only brings it up again

---

[1] We may here refer to the sensitive study of defiance by Th. Erismann in the periodical *Verstehen und Bilden*, 1. Jahrgang, 1926.

because of his visit to the pigeon. M. utilizes the opportunity afforded to point out that a pair of animals is necessary in order to produce offspring. The statement (*b*) shows that T. did not yet know this, or that he thought it of little importance and has forgotten it. He immediately draws the correct conclusion (*c*) from the information, that is, that Uncle P., a bachelor, will therefore have no children. J. has not grasped the matter, for he still thinks it possible for Uncle K. to have children (*d*), although he knows very well that he has no wife. Even in face of T's valid objection (*e*) J. still clings to the statement he has made (*f*).

132

5.10.27.   Evening in bed.

M. : " Julius, why don't you want any cod-liver oil to-day ? "

J. : " This tastes quite different."

M. : " Why, which do you like then ? "

T. : " Julius means quite different from the cake (which he is just eating).

M. : " Would you like a different kind of cod-liver oil ? "

J. : " Yes, German." (*a*).

T. : (Points to a label, on which two Easter Hares are represented) " Mama, why did Auntie O. draw a picture first ? I think she was so pleased with it when she'd done it that she drew another one at once. At first Auntie O. didn't even want to draw one, but then she drew two. Grandma, look, I think the Easter Hare has some peppermint-eggs, and you can eat them (*b*). Mama, when we were out for a walk we saw the Aunties (acquaintances of G.)."

G. : " Yes, we saw the Aunties."

T. : " When the memorial (War memorial) was being unveiled, we saw the Aunties then, and one of them was on the ladder."

J. : " The Aunties had a fine flag." (*c*).

T. : " It wasn't the old Auntie on the ladder, but the younger one, her sister."

J. : " They had visitors too."

T. : " Yes, you don't need to know one another there,

you just walk in (d). Mama, we were once in a week-end cottage (really about three weeks previously) and we sat in a summer house. We were allowed to, you hoped we could." (e).

J. : " Yes, it was fine in the summer house."

T. : " It's fine at the week-end cottage ; we should like to live there. Mama, why don't we build a house there ? " (f).

M. : " Yes, we could do that."

T. : " If you had plenty of money."

J. : " But if we already live here, we can't move, can we ? " (g).

T : (laughs out loud) " But Puschi moved, didn't she ? " (h).

J. : " But she's coming back again." (j).

T. : " No, she moved."

J. : " Why, did she hit you ? " (k).

T. : " No, she's not rude, she moved with the furniture van." (l).

J. : " But once, when you were small, she cried when she was with us." (m).

T. : " Only for a short time and then she stopped." (n).

J. : " Once Puschi opened the window wide." (o).

T. : " Then Mama called out. Why did you call out ? " (p).

M. : " For Minna to come and close the window. Children are not allowed at an open window, you know that."

T. : " Then Minna came and closed the window."

Discussion.—For the last three years as soon as the cold weather set in, children had been given doses of cod-liver oil until the spring. It was given in the form of the more palatable emulsion, and proved to be an excellent method of building up a healthy constitution. The children had a great liking for the emulsion, which they treated like a delicacy, and indeed they used to remind us of our duty in case we forgot to hand it out. From the very outset cod-liver oil had been praised in the children's hearing as something extremely good which would make them grow big and strong. Of course it must be suggested that it tastes very good, and the parents must never let it be suspected that they themselves would not like to take it. To-day was probably the first time that J. had refused to take cod-liver oil. It is possible that the contents of the bottle, which had been in use for several days, had become slightly rancid due to the warmer weather. The taste therefore may not have been quite so pleasant as usual, or it may be that T. was right in his suggestion that J. did not find the oil as tasty as the cake he was just eating, and so he refused it. When M. proposes " another " oil, and J. immediately decides for the " German " (*a*), he is only inventing a name to hide behind. We had never mentioned the fact that the cod-liver oil was not a German product. J. designates the previous oil as non-German, and therefore inferior, in order to justify himself in his own eyes and to triumph over his mother. He is degrading by name-magic what he has up till then considered good, in order to excuse his refusal to take it. Although in this case, by using the term " German " a good product is contrasted with an inferior or " non-German " one, this is merely invented for use on the spur of the moment and does not represent a general classification of value. For instance, all chocolate which the children wished to praise, irrespective of its real origin, was called " Swiss " chocolate. Stories about Switzerland which they had heard on occasion had surrounded everything connected with that country in a haze of glory. And so " Swiss " chocolate was superior to any other, and the most inferior brand was joyfully consumed if it had been introduced as " Swiss ". (*b*) The hares on the label had been roughly cut out by Auntie O. T. knows that G. likes peppermint tablets and so he lets one of the hares carry peppermint eggs, although nothing at all can be distinguished in the basket it is carrying. (*c*, *d*) The Aunties are owners of a small private hotel where G. had once stayed. A war memorial had been unveiled opposite to the hotel and it is to this that the children's remarks refer. In J's opinion the most important thing had been that the two Aunties had a fine flag. (*e*, *f*) Together with the children we had visited a week-end cottage not far from Rostock. The little house found so much approval that we now get the proposal to build a house there. (*g*) J.

thinks we could not move from our present house, probably because as yet he has never experienced a removal. He thinks we are fixed to our dwelling-place. (*h*) T. counters this quite correctly by pointing out that their former little friend Puschi removed too. The children had watched this removal, which had taken place some days previously with the closest attention. (*j*) J. thinks that Puschi will come back again, but T. explains once more that she has definitely removed. (*k*) Now comes a humorous misunderstanding. Instead of " moved " J. understands " rude ". T. corrects him (*l*), but J. will not own defeat so easily, and takes refuge in a very distant happening (*m*) when Puschi once was in tears. Weeping is not quite the same as being rude, it is true, but it lies in the same direction. (*n*) T. takes up the reference, but soon disposes of it. (*o*) J's thoughts take another leap and he brings up a dangerous situation in which the little friend found herself, one which is still a vivid memory to T. (*p*). The episode at the window ended by Puschi being taken away from her dangerous position by the maid, who came in when M. called out.

133

8.10.26. T. has accompanied his parents to the Psychological Institute. He is placing chairs in rows.

F. : (joking) " Are you going to give us a lecture ? "

M. : " We'll sit down and you'll lecture to us." (F. and M. sit down.)

T. : (takes the matter seriously and begins his lecture in an official tone of voice). " Ladies and Gentlemen, are you all here ? " (*a*).

F. and M. : " Yes, we're here."

T. : (in a lecturing voice) " Mother, your little daughter is foolish, she is so terribly childish." (From Tagore's *Waxing Moon*, from which M. had often read aloud to him. He can remember no more, and seeks fresh material.) " Once there went walking outside the door a coal-black Moor, the sun shone down upon his head and so he took a sunshade." (T. seeks new matter, but in spite of his obvious efforts, nothing occurs to him on the spur of the moment. His parents decided to release him from his uncomfortable situation.)

F. and M. : " Good, now we'll clap. The lecture was splendid." (T. puts the chairs away again. He appears to be quite satisfied with his first lecture.)

Discussion.—T. took the request for a lecture seriously. Just as in his other character plays he gets into a state of mind suited to the prevailing idea, so he does here. But whereas in all the previous parts he has played, the game was directed by amusement and fun, we notice on this occasion by his bearing and language that he is playing a serious part, and that the whole affair is serious, perhaps painfully serious to him. The introduction (*a*) is a reminiscence of Punch and Judy, and then the lecture proper begins. First of all he repeats with great emphasis a scrap of Tagore which has become fixed in his memory. Then he brings out a fragment of Struwelpeter. Whenever there was any mention of a lecture it seems as if T. had always understood it in the sense of the reproduction of some suitable material.

134

8.10.26. Evening in bed.

T. : " Mama, let us pray and talk." (*a*).

M. : " I'm coming."

T. : " Let us pray very softly."

J. : " I can pray alone."

T. : " Mama, you pray with me." (They do so.) " Mama from which ABC (book) is it easier to learn, from the Gardelegen one or the German ? Auntie O. thinks from the German. What do you think, tell me." (*b*).

M. : " It is just as easy in both. The children in Gardelegen learn more easily with their ABC book, and the Rostock children learn more easily from the Rostock book."

T. : " And in America ? " (*c*).

M. : " The children there learn easily from their own ABC."

T. : " Mama, you can't imagine how glad I am to have *Robinson Crusoe*." (*d*).

M. : " I'm very pleased that you are glad."

T. : " Mama, don't tell Auntie O. where *Robinson Crusoe* is, or she'll go and get it." (*e*).

M. : " Auntie O. will put it on the book shelf, she won't take it away from you."

T. : " *Robinson Crusoe* is a good book, isn't it ? " (*f*).

M. : " Yes, *Robinson Crusoe* is a very good book."

T. : " Are there other good books too ? " (*g*).

M. : " Later on you can read *Andersen's Fairy Tales*."

J. : " Andersen ? " (*h*).

T. : " It isn't the Danish boy Andersen, its an old man." (*j*).

M. : " Yes, this Andersen is a writer. The Danish boy who stayed with us wasn't a writer."

T. : " Mama, what other good books are there ? " (*k*).

M. : " *Uncle Tom's Cabin* is a very fine book."

T. : " I want that one, the Cabin, and what others are there besides ? " (*l*).

M. : " *The Good Comrade* " (a favourite German boy's annual).

T. : " Yes, that one too. I want all the books for my birthday." (*m*).

M. : " You can have some now, and others later on. You wouldn't be able to understand them yet."

T. : " Mama, did Robinson Crusoe really live ? " (*n*).

M. : " Yes. It often happens that people have to live on lonely islands and lead a life like Robinson Crusoe."

T. : " Some Spaniards came to Crusoe. Have Spaniards slanting eyes ? " (*o*).

M. : " No, they look just like we do."

T. : " Are they darker ? " (*p*).

M. : " Yes, you know that Uncle K. has been to Spain and he said you looked just like a little Spaniard. Now good night. Julius has already gone to sleep."

T. : " So go out very softly." (*q*).

M. : " Julius won't wake up. When he has fallen asleep he can't hear me going out."

T. : " No, but you disturb me." (*r*).

Discussion.—(*a*) Here for the first time T. mentions spontaneously in addition to praying also talking ; i.e. that chatting in a quite informal way which has become a necessity to him after he has prayed. (*b*) F. had brought back an ABC from a visit to a friend in Gardelegen. T. calls this the Gardelegen ABC and contrasts it with the Rostock ABC which he designates as " German ", meaning thereby " homely " and " familiar ". He has as yet no clear idea of what is German and what non-German. (*c*) It is clear that America has nothing to do with Germany from the fact that it can only be reached by ship. So T. thinks it possible that the state of affairs regarding ABC's may be quite different there. (*d*) His statement about Crusoe comes from the bottom of his heart. T. was almost beside himself with joy when he was recently given a copy of *Robinson Crusoe* for his own. Up till then he had heard the story read from a copy belonging to E. (*e*) T. jealously watches lest anyone should take the precious book from him. (*f, g, k, l, m*) These statements display a kind of literary interest which seems remarkable in a child not yet six years old. (*h, j*) We had once had visitors from Denmark, and among them a Mr. Anderson. Julius thinks that this acquaintance is possibly the author of fairy tales. T. is the first to discover J's mistake because he stands in closer contact with his brother's methods of thought than we adults, although he does not always make the same mistakes (conv. 18). (*m*) At first T. was probably quite convinced that Crusoe was a living person, but after he had been told so often with regard to fairy-tale characters " they didn't really live " he carries over this non-existence of people in stories to people who could or did actually exist. (*o, p*) T. is probably thinking of the Chinese, for he knows that they have slanting eyes, which he now applies generally as a criterion of strangeness. (*q, r*) These warnings are probably not to be taken seriously. They are phrases picked up and copied from adults, a practice which only rarely occurs in T. at this age. In reality T. was by no means the egoist intent on not being disturbed which he seems to be here.

135

9.10.26. Morning. The children come to their parents' beds. M. still has her eyes closed.

T.: "Mama, can you read some *Robinson Crusoe* to us ? "

M.: "No, I'm not properly awake yet. Go and lie down and try to sleep." (J. makes a noise.)

F.: "You must be quiet, Mama wants to sleep."

T.: "Julius be quiet."

J.: "I made a noise and Mama still didn't get up." (*a*).

T.: "It isn't a question of whether Mama gets up or not, it's a question of whether she can sleep or not." (*b*). (T. touches the lobe of F's ear.) "Papa, what are the lobes of the ear for ? " (*c*).

F.: "They're just there."

J.: "The lobes of the ears are there for washing." (*d*).

F.: (laughing) "You are clever, Julius."

J.: "Yes, I am clever." (Laughs.)

Discussion.—(*a, b*) Whereas J. still makes no difference between "sleeping " and " lying quiet with closed eyes " and considers as the opposite of both states being awake as " being up ", T. already has the necessary psychological insight to make this distinction. J's greater naïveté is also exemplified in the subsequent remarks (*c, d*). What are the lobes of the ears for asks T., just as an adult suddenly questions the right of existence of some thing or other which up to then, by reason of its very familiarity, has not presented any problems. The answer presents less difficulty to J. than to the adult. His answer probably contains two interpretations at once. J. means, the lobes are there in order to be washed. This definition is suggested by the fact that so much stress is laid on the daily ablutions ; the lobes of the ear must be clean too. But there is probably a second contributing factor also. The idea may have occurred to J. that the lobe of the ear has the same function as a dish-cloth (due to the similarity of sound between Ohrläppchen (lobe of the ear) and Waschläppchen (dish cloth). It is difficult for the adult to imagine these two ideas simultaneously, but the child finds no difficulty in effecting this fusion. Everyone from his own childhood will be able to remember examples of the possibility of such and even of more remarkable fusions of ideas, which the adult could not possibly perform. Of course there would have been no point in asking J. what was the meaning of his statement. That would have destroyed the naïveté of any explanation he might give. We may add in addition that T. discovered immediately how comical J's answer is. J. for his part recognizes from the prevailing hilarity that he has made some mistake, but welcomes the consolation and encouragement given by F.

136

10.10.26. Evening in bed.

J.: " Mama, I love you very much. Let us pray now. I'll pray first. I clasp my hands. I will be good. Now it's your turn." (a).

M.: " I will be good."

T.: " I will be good."

J.: " I will be good, I will not do anything naughty, Amen. Now I have said Amen."

M.: " Amen."

T.: " Amen."

M.: " Julius, have you been good to-day ? "

J.: " I must just think." (b).

T.: " I know already."

M.: " Theodor, just let Julius think."

J.: " I hit Theodor in the eye." (c).

T.: " Grandma said if Julius had had a knife in his hand it would have been worse."

J.: " If I had had a knife in my hand it would have been worse. Then I should have cut Theodor's eye out." (d).

M.: " You must never strike, Julius, or else something terrible may happen."

T.: " Mama, we threw the (gymnasium) rings so high that they went near the electric light. The lamp might have broken and we should all have been burned." (e).

J.: " That is nothing to laugh at." (f).

T. : " I'm not laughing, I'm sad too. They'd have to send for the fire brigade." (g).

J. : " I've seen all the fire brigade." (h).

T. : " And Mr. W's part (the landlord's apartments) might burn down too." (j).

J. : " Then we shall have to build another house, we shall have to go away." (k).

T. : " We can live with Auntie H., and it isn't so easy to go away, you have to pay for that, and the porter too, and all the things have to be packed up." (l).

J. : " Then we'll get some workmen in."

T. : " That's not so simple, you have to have a lot of money to do that."

M. : " Theodor, have you anything to tell me about what you have done to-day ? "

T. : " I will think about how it happened that Julius hit me to-day. Yes, I wanted to go out and Julius was going to give me the key, but he didn't want to and so I hit him with the shovel." (m).

M. : " With the iron shovel ? "

J. : " Theodor hit me on the body."

T. : " But Julius hit me worse." (n).

J. : " It's only a little place."

M. : " But it's in a dangerous place. Theodor might have lost his eye."

J. : " The iron shovel is more dangerous than the wooden one."

M. : " It's dreadful, I can't go out at all. I just have to stay in and watch you."

T. : " Oh do go out." (o).

M. : " But I have a husband and must be with him sometimes."

J. : " But you are more with your husband now." (p).

M. : " In Warnemünde I was with you all the time ; now I must be with Papa as well. Now let's go to sleep."

T. : " Mama, when you've had a little rest with us, you can go and learn some more." (p).

M. : " Yes, I'm looking forward to that. If only you once learn to read you'll read a great deal. You'll read aloud to Julius too."

J. : " I will learn to read, and read for myself." (r).

T. : " And then I can read a lot too." (s).

Discussion.—(*a*) J. seems to have the idea to-day that praying is a sort of party game, in which he is the " leader " whom all must follow. (*b*) J. knows very well what M. is hinting at, and is scarcely needing T's help to bring him to a confession of his impulsive misdemeanour (*c*). (*d*) To an adult it seems strange that J. can speak so coolly about an action which might have destroyed his brother's eye. Children of this age only feel pity for others when it is kindled in very specifically expressed forms, which are accessible to them. We see this also very clearly in the fact that children not only hear unmoved descriptions of the cruellest actions in fairy tales, but even express their approval. (*e*) T. makes spontaneously his own confession of sin which is connected with a strongly perseverative experience. And yet whilst describing the misdeed he cannot entirely conceal the glow of pleasure he felt in the game which the struggle provided. (*f*) T. was not laughing. We have here a phrase picked up from adults and used in the wrong place. (*g*) T. is not really sad. He probably means that he would have been sad had the affair had serious consequences. (*h*) For J. " fire brigade " is the cue to relate that he had seen the brigade driving through the streets, whilst T. brings the conversation back to the theme " fire " by stating (*j*) that if fire had broken out the house-owner's flat would have been in danger also. (*k, l*) Proposals in case the house had been burned down. (*m, n*) T. gives a calm and considered version of the dispute which had occurred between the two brothers. He tries to reconstruct the whole affair, exactly as if he were retelling the story in a court of law. He freely confesses that it was he who opened hostilities. On asking his grandmother we discovered that the whole affair had really proceeded just as described by T. (*o*) A fine example of T's self-sacrifice is shown here. T. recognizes that M. has a right to be together with F. occasionally, whereas J. maintains (*p*) (less because he has noticed it than to bolster up his own claims afresh) that M. is more with her " husband " now. (*q*) T. is referring to the fact that M. finds such great pleasure

in doing a little reading on scientific subjects after she has
finished attending to the children.   Here there is a clear
stirring of empathy into the wish-life of the mother.   (r) The
manly protest ! He refuses to be dependent on his brother,
and wants to be capable of providing for himself.   (s) Very
well, says T., in that case then I can read more for myself.

137

11.10.26.   At supper.
F. : " We saw a negro to-day."
T. : " Was he naked ? "
F. : " No, he was dressed."
J. : " In a bathing costume ? "
F. : " No, he was properly dressed."
J. : " He has rented a house I suppose."

Discussion.—To be a negro and to be naked is for the
children really one and the same thing.   Even if he was
dressed, then at the most in a bathing costume.   Why the
negro should have rented a house is difficult to see.

138

11.10.26.   Evening in bed.
T. : " Mama, are you going to bed now ? "
M. : " No, when you're asleep I'm going to learn a bit
more."
J. : " In a book as thick as this " (shows with his hands.)
T. : " It says in the book : ' Mother, your little daughter
is silly, she is so dreadfully childish.' "   (Cf. conv. 133.)
M. : " No, I'm not reading that book.   You know you
took it to Auntie G."
T. : " But Mama, then you won't have the book for your
lecture." (a).
M. : " Auntie G. will read it to-day and to-morrow she
will bring it back to me."
J. : " I shall cry when you go away."
M. : " You must not cry when I go away or I shall be
very sad."
J. : " I want you to stay with me always."
M. : " That cannot be.   But you mustn't cry, you must
get out of that habit."

J. : " How does one get out of a habit ? " (b).

M. : " You don't cry, give Mama a kiss and say good-bye and then Mama can go away happy."

T. : " I'm usually happy, but when Papa sings those sad songs about the war to me, then I get sad (c). Who made the war ? " (d).

M. : " All people together made the war."

T. : " Who began it ? " (e).

J. : " Perhaps the Kaiser ? " (f).

M. : " No."

T. : " When there's a war on, you can't get enough to eat and so you don't get big and strong (g). Mama, you've seen the Sultan, haven't you ? " (h).

M. : " I've seen the Kaiser too."

T. : " Where did you see the Kaiser ? "

M. : " In Berlin. Two officers rode past in a motor car and one of them saluted. That was the Kaiser."

T. : " Who was the other officer ? "

J. : " I suppose it was his warder ? " (j).

T. : " When did you see the Sultan ? "

M. : " When I was a little girl I was in Egypt with grandfather and grandmother and I saw the Sultan there, but I don't remember very much about it."

J. : " Tell half then." (k).

M. : " The carriage had to drive slowly."

J. : " Yes, so that it didn't buffer." (l).

T. : " Did you go and meet the Sultan ? "

M. : " No, I only saw him drive past."

T. : " Lots of people are lucky and are let in (m). Let us pray now, but very softly."

M. : " Have you anything to tell me ? "

J. : " Yes, Papa did frighten me. When G. opened the door he jumped out suddenly."

M. : " Papa was only playing. Theodor, have you anything to tell me ? "

T. : " No, I can't think of anything to-day."

M. : " Were you kind to Grandma ? "

T. : " Yes."

M. : " But you said to Grandma ' bad night ' instead of ' good night '."

T. : " I won't do that again." (n).

P

Discussion.—(*a*) T. means M's lecture at the Volkshochschule where M. occasionally read excerpts from Tagore. (*b*) At times J. is almost beside himself when his parents go out together or when M. goes out alone. His question as to how one can rid oneself of this habit of crying, although it strikes us as comical, is meant quite seriously by J. (*c*) An outsider will scarcely be able to trace out how T. arrives at this statement. It is caused by the " good-bye " (Wiedersehen). F. had recently sung several songs to the children, and one of these had the chorus " We shall see each other in the homeland " (In der Heimat da gibts ein Wiedersehen). This song had made T. sad, probably more because of its tune than its words. No other sad war-songs had been sung. (*d, e*) It is a sign of a good capacity for thinking that T. distinguishes between those who made the war and those who began it. (*f*) We need not say that J. had never heard anything at home about the Kaiser having begun the war. But to J. the Kaiser is such an impressive, important personality that he must take precedence here, as he did in all other circumstances, and so he must have begun the war. (*g*) Just as in conversation 19, we see here too that what T. had heard about the scarcity of food during the war had made a deep impression on him. (*h*) The Sultan is undoubtedly called forth by the mention of the Kaiser. (*j*) This means " the man who is responsible for the Kaiser's safety ". (*k*) How simple is J's conception of emotional circumstances. If one can no longer remember the whole, then at least perhaps the half, and M. shall tell them this. (*l*) " Buffer " is a splendid invention. He means of course so that the carriage shall not come into collision. (*m*) T. has forgotten that the meeting with the Sultan took place in the street. He connects the Sultan with his Palace and asks if M. were admitted into the Palace. (*n*) T. had wished Grandma " Bad night " instead of " Good night ". Certainly he did not mean this maliciously, but on the spur of the moment he just could not resist the idea which thrust itself upon him associatively. He had no conception of the meaning of the nightly greeting. He recognizes this now, and is sorry, as we see from his own statement.

139

12.10.26. Evening in bed.

T. : " Mama, I've not heard anything of *Robinson Crusoe* the whole day. You must read some of it to me." (*a*).

M. : " I can't now, it's late already." (M. closes her eyes.)

J. : " Theodor, Mama is asleep." (*b*).

T. : " Mama, you are tired."

J. : " Softly, Mama wants to sleep. She can't read now, she'll ruin her eyes." (*c*).

T. : " Mama must not read in the dark. She ought to switch on the reading lamp." (*d*).

M. : " Theodor, if you want to hear about *Robinson Crusoe* go to the nursery and ask Auntie O. to read to you."

T. : " I'll bring *Crusoe* here. Mama, switch on the light."

J. : " I'll switch the light on, Mama. The little brother must of course always switch on the light for his big brother." (J. switches on the light, T. brings *Robinson Crusoe*.) (*e*).

J. : " Theodor, you read." (*f*).

T. : (opening the book) " Once there was a man called Robinson Crusoe who was shipwrecked on an island where he built a house, then he met a lama, then he met Friday, then Friday brought his father, then they sailed away. Mama, you read now." (*g*).

J. : " But you were reading yourself." (*h*).

T. : " No, I wasn't reading, I was only pretending to read." (*j*).

J. : " Mama, shall I say something ? " (*k*).

M. : " Yes, say everything that you have to say."

J. : " There once was a man
He went to the strand
And there ate bread and sand." (*l*)

M. : " Children, have you anything to tell me ? "

J. : " But we haven't prayed yet. First we must pray and then we can talk. I'll pray first." (M. and T. pray with him.) " I will be good. . . . " (*m*).

J. : " Amen."

M. and T. : " Amen."

M. : " Have you anything to tell me now ? "

T. : " I know what J. has to tell." (*n*).

M. : " Theodor, J. knows what he will say."

J. : " When Papa and Mama wanted to go out I was naughty and cried, only for a moment, and then I stopped." (*o*).

T. : " It was longer than a moment."

J. : " It was a minute." (*p*).

T. : " It was many minutes."

M. : " Julius, but now you know that Mama must go out with Papa, and you won't cry."

J. : " Yes Mama, you must go out, you must have fresh air or else you'll die." (*q*).

M. : " Theodor, have you anything to tell me ? "

T. : " When you and Papa were going out I told Julius." (*r*).

M. : " Was that good or naughty ? "

T. : (Rather defiantly) " Good." (*s*).

M. : " But you made Julius sad ; just think whether that was good or naughty."

Discussion.—(*a*) " Diem perdidi ". A day when nothing of *Robinson Crusoe* was read aloud was a wasted day. (*b*) Wild and boisterous as J. could frequently be, yet he showed great concern whenever he noticed that M. was tired and exhausted. This is expressed in his further remark (*c*). (*d*) T. means that it is only reading in the dark which makes M. so tired, and therefore the light should be switched on. (*e*) The principle J. lays down, which, by the way, he himself has formulated, is probably not the real motive of his action, but the joy in the act of switching on the light itself. He would probably scarcely have been so ready to perform a less diverting action, even for the sake of the principle. (*f*) J. thinks that T. can read already, for he has been having reading lessons for some days now. (*g*) T. pretends to read aloud. What he reproduces of the book is characteristic of his conception of *Robinson Crusoe* : he gives the most thrilling episodes. (*h*) We see that J. has already taken T's reading aloud seriously, whereas T. points out the humorous element (*j*). Now J. would like to " say something " (*k*) by which he means inventing rhymes. (*l*) A sample of his muse. (*m*) J. feels troubled because prayers have not yet been said. He prays first, just as in conversation 136. (*n*) T. wants to bring forward the main sin J. has committed on this day, or at least he makes it clear that he knows what J. has to confess. (*o*) J. knows very well what it is about. He had protested violently when the parents were setting out for a walk. To diminish his guilt he maintains that the whole affair only lasted a minute (*p*) although of course he has no accurate conception of the extent of a minute. (*q*) J. recognizes that he ought not to prevent M. from going out, but he exaggerates the ill effects of house air. (*r, s*) T. had drawn J's attention to the fact that the parents were going out, otherwise he would not have noticed it. That was very wrong of him, because by this means he upset J. However, it is probable that the real motive of his action did not occur to him clearly.

140

14.10.26. At table. The children had seen the " Frog King " at the theatre the previous day.

F. : " You are my little Frog King."

J. : " And I'll tie a tree round me " (probably he means a branch) " and say that is my sword, and tie a pear on my head and say that is my crown. Do frogs like potatoes ? "

F. : " No, frogs eat flies."

J. : " Yes, but the frog in the theatre didn't eat any flies."

F. : " Because there weren't any flies there."

J. : " The man who has possession (!) of the theatre ought to make some flies." (*a*).

F. : " Next time you're at the theatre tell the man he ought to have some flies flying about."

J. : " Mama, why was the frog so big ? "

M. : " It was a man dressed as a frog."

T. : " Who threw the ball into the water ? "

M. : " Do you know, Julius ? "

J. : " No."

M. : " The page threw the ball into the water."

T. : " Has the king's daughter always a fountain ? "

M. : " Yes, the king's daughter in the Frog King always has a fountain."

J. : " I knew at once that it was the park."

T. : " Julius, you can't know everything, you don't even know your ABC." (b).

J. : " How does the ABC go ? "

T. : " ABC, the cat sees me." (c).

J. : " I can count too."

T. : " Oh you, that's not counting. How did they make the king ? " (d).

M. : " Do you want to know how they made the king in the theatre ? "

T. : " No, how they used to make him always."

M. : " They always used to elect the most able man. He ruled the people and gave them advice."

T. : " What does ' elect ' mean ? " (e).

M. : " Everyone writes a name on a slip of paper, F, M, G, O, or E. If everyone writes Theodor, then you're ' elected '. What do you think Julius, who ought to be king ? "

J. : " I."

T. : " No, Papa. But what happens if different names are written ? " (f).

M. : " Then the one is elected whose name is written most often."

T. : " Mama, what does ' advice ' mean ? " (g).

M. : " If for instance you have a dispute about your cart, you go to the king and the king gives you the advice to play alternately with the cart."

J. : " And if I have asked him, and Theodor doesn't give me the cart and says I haven't one ? "

M. : " The people who have elected the king obey him too."

T. : " I got a fright when the crash came (when the Frog King was freed from the spell)." (h).

J. : " Do you know what I thought ? His heart was breaking."

T. : " Why was the Frog King so sad ? "

M. : " Because the witch had cast a spell on him."

J. : " But we didn't see a witch who cast a spell on the frog."

T. : " Why do we see the shadows in the theatre ? " (*j*).

M. : " Everywhere where there is illumination a shadow results."

T. : " Oh yes."

M. : " Have you ever watched your shadow ? "

T. : " Yes, I've seen my shadow too. Why could not Henry say what he was changed into (i.e. the Prince) ? " (*k*).

M. : " Henry could not say because otherwise the prince would always have remained a frog."

T. : " Did he really not like it (i.e. did the actor like being bewitched) ? (*l*). Why did the pate (page) attack the frog ? "

M. : " That was very rude of the page."

T. : " But the king did not attack the frog, did he ? "

M. : " No, you know the frog was the king's guest. It is just as if you invited Anke B. to come and see you and then attacked her."

J. : " But we can set about Wilhelm B. (Anke's brother) ? "

M. : " If he gives you permission to do so."

T. : " What does ' permission ' mean ? "

M. : " ' Permission ' means, if Wilhelm B. says ' attack me '. Then he has given you permission."

T. : " I suppose there was a boy in the frog dress ? A grown-up would surely not have allowed the pate (!) to jump on him." (*m*).

J. : " The page girl (the page had a girlish appearance and was indeed played by an actress) was very rude, wasn't she ? "

T. : " Mama, is it nicer in the cinema than in the theatre ? " (*n*).

M. : " It is much nicer in the theatre. In the theatre are living people and fine stories."

T. : " Are there no stories in the cinema ? "

M. : " Yes, but they are told in pictures."

T. : " Can one look at the pictures as long as one likes ? "

M. : " No, the pictures are only shown for a short time. An uncle photographed you when you were playing in Warnemünde. That is a picture just as at the cinema."

T. : " Can you hear what we say too ? " (*o*).

M. : " No, we can't hear what you say."

T. : " Is October over yet ? " (*p*).

M. : " No, only half. Your birthday is on 8th November."
(M. closes her eyes.)

J. : (seeing M.) " Theodor, Mama is dead." (*q*).

T. : " Mama." (*r*).

M. : " Yes, Theodor."

T. : " Mama, when I heard you speak, I know that you are not dead." (*s*).

M. : " No, I was only tired and closed my eyes. If one has closed one's eyes, one isn't immediately dead. When we are asleep we always have our eyes closed."

Discussion.—As can be seen from their subsequent remarks, the children had been able to follow the action of the Frog King : T. completely and J. almost completely. (*a*) For J. the illusion is much more powerful and so he demands for the frog the food it needs. (*b*) T. parades his newly acquired knowledge in order to triumph over J., although he too does not know very much about it (*c*). (*d*) With the spontaneous theme " king " the conversation takes a new turn. T's skilful questions about the principles of an election in general and of a king in particular are worthy of note (*e, f, g*). After this business has been disposed of, T. comes back again to the theatre with his remark (*h*). Question (*j*) reveals his good observation. After this theoretical question has been answered he again returns to the play, with question (*k*). This constant returning to the main theme after going into subsidiary questions arising in the course of the conversation takes place purely perseveratively. Perseveration acts here with the effect of a most gratifying discipline of the course of conversation. (*l*) This complete fusion of actor and his part, and the corresponding confusion of feelings often happens even to an uneducated adult at the theatre. In (*m*) too there is revealed a similar confusion. It is not quite clear to T. that the actor is playing a part and cannot adopt an attitude dictated by his own personal feelings. (*n*) T. has as yet only heard about the cinema and has no proper conception of this institution. (*o*) The children had been photographed on the beach with a baby-ciné camera, but had not themselves seen the film.   Here T. has the idea of a talkie. (*p*) The conversation takes another new turn.   T. is hinting at his birthday. (*q*) We see quickly how, even at J's age, the declaration of death takes place, and not only quickly, but in a very cool and matter-of-fact way.   (*r*) T. is not a little shocked by this announcement of death, and is very glad (*s*) to discover an important criterion of life in M.

141

20.10.26.   Evening in bed.

J. : " Mama, I am so afraid."

M. : " What are you afraid of ? "

J. : " I can't tell you or else you'll be afraid too." (*a*).

M. : " Don't be afraid to tell me, I'm not afraid of anything."

T. : " Not even of a rhinoceros ? " (*b*).

M. : " I don't care a rap for a rhinoceros."

T. : " Then it will run away, won't it ? " (*c*).

J. : " But I am so afraid." (*d*).

M. : " What are you afraid of ? Of a witch ? You know there aren't any, people have only imagined them."

J. : " No."

M. : " Of devils ? There aren't any of those either."

J. : " No, Mama you know there are no longer any of those. What are those ' claves ' ? " (*e*).

M. : " Perhaps you mean slaves ? "

J. : " Yes, they beat with whips." (*f*).

T. : " No, they don't beat with whips, they are beaten with whips." (*g*).

M. : " There aren't any slaves now."

J. : " But I dream about them." (*h*).

T. : " Close your eyes. Do you see any slaves now ? " (*j*).

J. : " No."

T. : " You see, then you have no vibratory sense (*k*). Mama, what is instinct ? " (*l*).

M. : " When a chicken is born, it immediately begins to peck food, then we say it has instinct."

J. : " Mama, has everybody instinct ? " (*m*).

M. : " Yes, everybody eats by instinct."

T. : " Mama, do you think it is called that because it stinks ? " (*n*).

M. : " No, it has nothing to do with that."

Discussion.—(*a*) It does not seem as if J. at this moment is feeling much fear, and perhaps he only means that he is afraid when he thinks of the things spoken about later on. He fears M. may also be attacked by fear of the same thing and so will not inform her about what he fears so much. (*b*) T. thinks M. has been too quick in declaring her fearlessness, and that she might indeed be afraid of a rhinoceros. We cannot say why T. should think of just this animal. It is possible that special mention had been made of the ferocity of this animal in one of the hunting stories recently read to him. (*c*) T. takes the ' rap ' literally and interprets it as being used to scare away the animal. (*d*) J. returns perseveratively to his fear, and now it appears (*e*) that " claves " (he means slaves) are the object of his fear. (*f*) The slaves owe their fearsomeness to a misunderstanding of the child. He has understood the stories about slaves to say that they beat other people, but T. corrects him (*g*) by explaining that they themselves are beaten. (*h*) Probably J's fear of slaves is not based on a dream or dreams, but on the fact that he has been concerned with them in his imagination. (*j*) How simple is T's method of convincing his younger brother of the non-existence of the slaves. If J. sees no slaves when he closes his eyes, then there are none. The conclusion drawn by T. that J. has no vibratory sense (*k*) (conv. 51) certainly goes too far. (*l*) T. has already an understanding for things which are psychologically connected. From the vibratory sense he proceeds to the question about instinct. (*m*) J's question is probably not meant in a deeper sense. (*n*) The question is indeed justified by the similarity in sound.

PART II : GENERAL RESULTS

I. CHARACTEROLOGY

Anyone considering the utterances of the two children (as given in the foregoing conversations) from the point of view of their personal note, would at once be struck by the fact that the outlines of two quite distinct childish individualities are revealed. Those differences of attitude towards environment, which are determined by a difference in age, are easily distinguishable from those which are to be attributed to differences in their dispositions, that is their character and temperament. Of course the existing difference in age cannot be excluded experimentally, but the earliest recorded utterances of Theodor can be compared with those of Julius occurring later in the conversations. By this means we can place side by side utterances of the children when they were both about the same age (conversation recorded subsequently will make possible accurate comparisons with no difference in age intervening) and by this means we discover the utter hopelessness of the assumption that differences in age alone are to be made use of in explaining differences in appraising environment. No, through all the changes which are revealed as a consequence of intellectual development in the utterances of the two children as their age increases, we see developing two distinct childish personalities, which however remain identical in their development. There are fragments of conversation which have so neutral a tint that they might have originated from either of the two children or even from other children of the same age, but in all the conversations where evaluations have to be made (and these constitute the great majority) the personality behind the scenes discloses itself and the conversations belong to the children just as do their features and their physical make-up. The object of this section is to sketch the two childish personalities from their conversations and by making use of further material noted in our scientific diaries. This task has, so far as we know, scarcely ever been undertaken in the available literature of child psychology, apart from the attempt of E. Köhler.[1] In this section elements of character, i.e. individual characteristics are to be brought out, whereas in the subsequent sections we shall attempt to give the characterization a more general application.

Characterological observations have already been made at various points in individual conversations and our task is now to round these off properly. In order to do this we shall adopt the same plan as before, i.e. we shall demonstrate the development by comparing the two brothers with each other in order to get at their difference. For the process of absolute characterization in a subject like child psychology where as yet so little is known about the main characterological guiding principles—in so far as one can speak of any guiding principles—is fraught with special dangers. At what age does the character of children begin to become scientifically tangible ? At least from the moment when the child adopts some attitude towards its social environment ; but there is ample opportunity much earlier than this to determine other individual differences. In view of the great importance attached to human physical characteristics by modern characterology (investigation is strongly influenced by Kretschmer [2]) it may be of value to give some information about the physical constitution of the two boys. If the physical characteristics of T. and J. are compared, it is easy to note quite definite differences between them. Taking as our basis photographs of the children taken at the same age, we notice that T. is much slimmer and more

---

[1] " No one as yet has dared to try . . . to shape completely in all its detail a child's individuality development." W. Stern, *Differentielle Psychologie*, 3rd ed., Leipzig, 1921.

[2] E. Kretschmer : *Körperbau und Charakter*. 5. u. 6. Ed. Berlin 1926.

muscular than his brother, who is built on more massive, squat lines. In spite of an excellent appetite and the best nourishing food T. has never been able to put on flesh, whilst J., under the same conditions, has acquired a certain rotundity and accumulation of fat. T's tendency to slimness and J's plumpness is revealed not only on body and limbs but is even repeated on fingers and toes, both of which are particularly slim in T's case. One might dare to say with all cautiousness that T. inclines towards the asthenic and J. towards the pyknic type. In this respect T. has inherited his characteristics from his grandfather on his mother's side and J. from his grandfather on his father's side. Other physical characteristics of the two boys also seem to belong to this sphere of inheritance. T. has brown eyes, straight brown hair, and brownish pigmentation of the skin ; J. has greyish-blue eyes, slightly curly hair and a skin with very slight pigmentation. To us parents and also to strangers the children seem to have very little resemblance to each other.

The expressive movements of the two children are very different. At the same age T. was more graceful and supple in his movements than was J. It was comparatively rare for T. to fall down clumsily, and even when he did he escaped almost always without damage. When J. was the same age he was on much more familiar terms with Mother Earth, and could always display some scar or bruise, which, however, he never took seriously. It cannot be said that J. was more daring in his behaviour than T., but the latter's greater skill saved him oftener from falling when for instance during play the two boys had climbed on rickety structures of their own contrivance. Occasionally T. would jump from such heights that we as parents had to raise vigorous protests.

Both children have happily been spared serious illness up to the present, and J. has been freer than T. from slight indisposition. J. suffered remarkably little from a slight attack of whooping-cough ; many children are very distressed by the fits of coughing and lose weight perceptibly.

But J. on the contrary not only suffered no loss of weight but even increased it a little, which is proof positive of a fundamentally healthy constitution. It may be of interest for the investigation of the correlation between a child's physical constitution and his susceptibility to infectious disease to mention quite emphatically that T. remained quite immune from infection by whooping-cough, even though he was in contact with his brother in the normal way.

T. got accustomed to habits of cleanliness much earlier than J., and in fact our general impression is that cleanliness of body, clothing, and finally of food became for him a much greater necessity than they ever did for his younger brother. T. would very rarely touch any article of food with dirty hands, and after he had once been informed that he should not eat food dropped on the ground, he kept quite strictly to this rule, which cannot be said of J., who is extremely loath to let a tasty morsel lie on the ground. Up to the present J. has retained a decided tendency to put objects with which he is playing into his mouth. This is due to a habit of sucking which he acquired very early, in all probability not without the kind assistance of an incorrigible nursemaid he had at the time. T. has never had this sucking habit.

In several individual discussions on appetite we have already given hints of the differences in the children's preferences. We will summarize what has already been said and amplify it by further examples. Reduced to a brief formula : T. is inclined towards a vegetarian mode of life ; indeed to such a degree that in this direction his taste clearly differs from the average kind of food usual for children at this time. On the other hand J. is almost, if not quite, equally removed from the average in the other direction, that is towards the enjoyment of meat. The following may be added to what has already been demonstrated in the conversations about the children's favourite dishes and their food in general. T. used to drink the milk of coco-nuts with extreme pleasure ; in this it is quite probable that in addition to the immediate sensory pleasure there was present the ideal one that coco-nuts and their milk played such an important part in the diet of the adored *Robinson Crusoe*. The romantic aspect of this source of milk, together with the tendency to imitation, caused J. too, to ask for some of the juice, but he only tasted it and then disappointedly abandoned the remainder at once to his brother, who was looking on with longing eyes. We have previously stated that T. had a far greater liking for fruit than J. The only exception to this rule which we have as yet noticed is the locust, which J. eats ravenously, whereas it is refused by T. It must, however, be admitted that locust in consistency and taste is not specifically fruit-like but rather like a sweetish bread, as the name St. John's Bread implies. And with regard to the meat diet of the children it has been revealed that T. only ate lean meat, while J. preferred the fatty portions and even consumed pure fat with great delight.

Concerning the children's drink, both children, up to a few months before the conclusion of this work, had known only milk and cocoa as a means of quenching thirst. Only recently have they begun to quench their thirst with water, very weak tea or raspberry water. As this took place at the same time for both boys, it would have been expected that T. would be the first to give up the childish enjoyment of milk, but exactly the opposite was the case, for J. turned to the new beverages with greater liking and one day declared that water and fruit juice was certainly the best drink. Can it be an accident that it was easier for J. to give up milk, the basic drink ? Or is this not connected with his physical constitution ? Let us put the question in the general form : Are there any inner relations between a person's physical constitution and the direction of his appetite ?

So far as we know there are available no investigations into this subject so far as adults are concerned ; but even if there were, when we consider the numerous proved experiences about alterations in the direction of taste due to the influence of custom, it is obvious that they would demand completion by means of observations made on children. One need only think of the so-called traditional aversion to certain foods, which, for instance, makes the enjoyment of rotten eggs intolerable for West Europeans, whereas in other quarters of the globe they are accounted a great delicacy. This reveals that it is certain that a great many of our food likes and dislikes are not radical, but determined by the influences of education.   Discoveries made in the nursery, if noted carefully, offer some prospect of gaining an insight into the natural tendency of taste and so into its variations as dependent on the physical constitution.

In accordance with the generally accepted view that a vegetarian diet is more suitable for children in their earliest years than one containing meat, we introduced into the nursery a diet which was principally vegetarian. The two children behaved selectively towards the same diet, T. showing a decided preference for the vegetarian dishes and J. an equally strong preference for those containing meat. Thus the experiment has something of the strictness and accuracy of an experimental process.   The method of preparation of the dishes served was of course relatively haphazard, and it must be assumed that the appetite is less concerned with seeking a dish prepared in a special way, than with finding definite foods which the organism and the individual organism needs.   This was shown particularly clearly by those foods (e.g. most kinds of fruit) which the children ate raw.   The differing directions of appetite observed in our children can scarcely be fortuitous, but appear to be rooted in the varying requirements of their bodies. It is probably not going too far to say that they are connected with their differing physical constitutions. One might almost say it appears " understandable ", that J's more robust body would lead us to expect him to prefer a heavier diet, rich in albumen and fats, while T's more slender figure is more in harmony with lighter foods containing starch and sugar. It might also appear understandable that J. should be always the greater realist at table and more interested than his brother in ample supplies of good though simple food. But we do not wish to add another misuse to the already heavy list connected with the terms " understand ". If there really do exist between the physical constitution of the child and the direction of his appetite connections of the kind we believe we have succeeded in discovering here, then it is not a question of a connection governed by structural laws, but of a purely empirical-causal connection. The probability of the connection is determined by the extent to which our discoveries are confirmed by statistics in future investigations.[1]

It is probably one of the most remarkable functions of the psychological organism, that the psychological need reveals itself in the form of an appetite for definite foods or dishes, by means of which the need can be supplied. Through all the disguises imposed on foods by the cooks of various countries and nations the appetite succeeds in extracting from the dishes those components which the body needs, as Rubner for instance proved in his researches.[2] Apart from experiments on animals, experiments and observations on children have the best prospects of succeeding in obtaining an insight into the circumstances surrounding appetite.[3]

The traditional aversion to food occurs usually as a result of the condemnation of certain dishes or foods on the authority of adults.[4] The resultant socially-determined taboo in the sphere of food is quite different from the

---

[1] This connection is therefore not in the sense in which Erismann uses the word, intelligent (*einsichtig*) but " it just is so ". Th. Erismann, *Die Eigenart des Geistigen*, Leipzig, 1924.

[2] Of the numerous works on this subject we mention only M. Rubner, " Der Nahrungstrieb des Menschen," *Sitzungsberichte der Preussischen Akademie der Wissenschaften*, Berlin, 1920.

[3] Cf. D. Katz, *Hunger und Appetit*, Leipzig, 1932.

[4] Julian Hirsch, " Ueber traditionellen Speiseabscheu," *Zeitschr. f. Psychol.*, vol. 88, 1922.

aversion to foods, which develops in the child without or even against the wishes of adults. We may quote the following example. Our children have a distaste for all fish dishes amounting to an aversion. This aversion we have noticed for about a year, during which time the children have refused even to sit at a table where there was a fish dish, even though it was not meant for them. If they are, however, compelled to sit at table, they either look away from the fish or keep their eyes closed, so that they do not see it. Endowed with a very keen sense of smell, the children very quickly discover when fish is being prepared in the kitchen. It is not possible to say with certainty how this aversion to fish arose, for it would be one of the last things to expect of children living near the sea coast. The probability is that it originated in T., who perhaps disliked both the appearance and the smell of dead fish, and that J. then proceeded to adopt the aversion from his elder brother. If for any reason an aversion to a food has once been formed in a child the person undertaking its training has to choose between two courses. Shall he let the child omit the dish concerned at table, or shall he insist that the child should overcome its loathing ?

In general the question is not easy to answer. We have tried never to compel the children to eat fish dishes, and we have very little sympathy with compulsion in these matters, so long as the aversion to certain dishes does not give the impression of being due to pure fastidiousness.[1]

We here include a number of observations about hunger and thirst as the motives of action in the child, which may possibly be of general importance. The child announces that it is thirsty very much oftener than that it is hungry, or more precisely, it makes a spontaneous demand for drink much more frequently than for food.[2] When the children

---

[1] St. Engel also declares against any compulsion. *Schlecht essende Kinder. Monatsschrift fuer Kinderheilkunde*, vol. 30.

[2] Biologically thirst has in every respect a prior claim over hunger. The torments of thirst are worse than those of hunger, and Tantalus was tormented with thirst. Behind the powerful urge to quench thirst we perceive the importance of water in the economy of the living substance

woke in the morning, or (if they had been sleeping), in the afternoon, they habitually asked for milk and each used to drink at a draught about half a pint. Later on the milk could be replaced by some other drink which then had the same thirst-quenching effect. The desire for drink is expressed without any liquid being at the time visible in the child's surroundings. The feeling of thirst is so strong that it is able to call up the means of its removal by means of ideas into the child's consciousness. The conditions seem to be rather different in the case of hunger. A child may be extremely hungry, as it shows by eating an unusually large amount of food, and yet even in such a state it does not always make a spontaneous demand for food, unless it catches sight of food, or unless the situation (laying the table, preparations in the kitchen, smell of the food being prepared, etc.) calls up the idea of food. Our children could play for hours at a time without taking any solid food. Then, when they came to table, it was clear from the amount they consumed how greatly their bodies had really needed nourishment. Doubtless in such cases there exists a subjective feeling of hunger, but without external help, such as is afforded for instance by the sight of food, this feeling is not as easily converted into a demand for the means of appeasing hunger as the feeling of thirst is into a demand for means to quench the thirst. Very much greater states of hunger must be reached to cause a spontaneous demand for food to be made. As evidence of this we include the following example from our diary.

15.1.24. T. was living on a very restricted diet because of an attack of diarrhœa. He was given nothing but tea and a few biscuits. When F. came home in the evening of 15.1.24. T. greeted him with " What have you brought for me ? Eggs and rice ? " Usually he is by no means so interested in such things and asks for chocolate, cakes or sweets. When he awoke on 16th January he said to his mother : " Give me some carrots and potatoes with gravy, and some pudding with fruit juice." Thus T. had gone over the whole of his usual menu, a thing which in normal circumstances he never did in the morning, when he usually asked only for milk or cocoa. It had required two days of starvation to awaken, at a most unusual time, the desire for food, and, as we see, for very substantial food.

The following case also shows that feelings of hunger seem to be bound complexly to definite situations much more in children than in adults. On a school excursion a five-year-old boy who had been taken by his brother, strayed from the rest of the class and could not be found in the evening when it was time to return. The child remained undiscovered the whole night and until the next afternoon. Then he was found by school children who had been mobilized in the quite justified belief that the little boy might perhaps keep out of the way of adults searching for him. Then the remarkable discovery was made that the child still had with him the sandwiches packed for him by his mother. They were untouched, although the child must have been famished by his twenty-four hours' fast. When his mother asked him why he had not eaten the sandwiches, the child replied that he had been told to eat them when he was in the tram on the homeward journey. It could therefore be said that in obedience to his mother's advice, which he had taken for a binding order, the child had not even touched the sandwiches, in spite of an extreme feeling of hunger. But we should prefer to assume that the child, removed from his usual routine, was not so acutely conscious of hunger as usual, as the corresponding situations had now disappeared. In any case chance carried out here a very remarkable experiment in child psychology and one which is worthy of notice from more than one point of view.

We will now briefly discuss the question of the behaviour of the children towards animals. This theme has already been touched on in (6).[1] J. will go up to strange dogs in the street, even the larger ones, and stroke them. T. would

---

[1] A figure in parentheses indicates here and afterwards the conversation concerned.

never do this, even when encouraged by us, as he really has a definite fear of dogs. We can amplify this statement by other observations along similar lines. We were keeping a few white mice in the Psychological Institute for experimental purposes and the children once paid them a visit. J. immediately seized the little creatures without any fear or aversion and laughingly let them run over his hands, delighted with their tricks. It did not trouble him whether he pulled the mice from their nest by their heads or their tails. T., who was following the antics of the animals with rapt attention would not himself have touched the animals for anything in the world. Indeed he called out several times when he saw that J. was handling the creatures so unceremoniously. On other occasions too T. was concerned when he thought that a member of the family was handling animals too carelessly. The following observations shows how little J. himself was affected in his subsequent behaviour by an unfortunate experience with an animal to which he had taken a liking. J. was playing at home with the rabbit which played the part of the Easter Hare at Easter time. Whilst he was trying to push some food into the animal's mouth, the rabbit, not understanding his kind intention, bit one of his fingers so deeply that it bled and F. had to bandage it up. Without any further ado J. immediately approached the animal with his bandaged finger. Obviously the behaviour of children towards animals is determined much less by good and unpleasant experiences with animals than by a disposition which is quite original. T. is extremely interested in animals and he likes them, but it is a liking from a distance. He is by nature shy of contact with animals, whilst J. tries to fondle every animal he can get hold of. We may judge how strong this tendency in him is from the fact that even the negative example set by T. has not been able to do it any serious harm. Timidity towards animals does not by any means justify us in assuming general timidity. In the gymnasium and elsewhere T. exposes his body to no less risks than J.

What children see in animals, or respectively what they see into them, is important characterologically. T. makes the monkeys he saw at the Zoo behave in a decent human way, whereas, J. understands their actions as " playing tricks " (73). J. also makes the monkeys in the Institute play tricks and get into mischief, for that coincides with his conception of the use an animal would like to make of its unrestrained freedom (77). From these and similar observations about the understanding which children have of the expressive movements and behaviour of animals, it has been revealed that the interpretation depends to a great extent on the mental disposition of the person interpreting.[1] In general we may say that children assume their own likes and desires to be present in adults. The presents for the father (129) are decided according to the child's tastes.

Of the two brothers J. is the greater egoist, although probably he is not more attentive to his own interests than the average child of his own age. But on the other hand it is almost certain that T. excels the usual child of his age in self-sacrifice and self-renunciation. It is very difficult to induce J. to give up a share of any dainty, once he has become possessed of it, whereas T. is just the reverse and gives up things easily (110). T. has the greater capacity for empathy, he inquires about the fate of other people and is concerned about their troubles and difficulties. He does not like to hear that other people are suffering hardships, whilst J. is very little affected by such matters. Here too J's behaviour probably approximates more closely to the normal, whilst T's capacity for sympathy is in advance of his years. T. is sad that his father has gone away, whilst J. finds consolation in the fact that a humorous letter from him will arrive : this is for him a completely satisfactory substitute for his father's absence (40). When the father

---

[1] We are investigating the question of the interpretation by children of expressive movements of animals. Perhaps the investigation will clear up some points about the genesis of certain forms of understanding.

playfully pretends to be dumb, J. only finds it comical, whilst T. becomes perturbed (128). Soldiers' songs, sentimental in the melody, rather than in the text, make T. sad (138). If J. jokingly attacks his father, T. rushes in to the defence of his parents and seems concerned about a danger to his father which in reality had never existed at all. When the father returns from a journey J. is ready to play a trick on him, but T. is horrified at the idea, and this is probably not merely because he is afraid of forfeiting the presents, but because he simply does not want to play a trick on his father (118). The two children differ in their type of empathy towards other people including people represented in pictures. Both children look at Dürer's " Melancholie ". T. asks why the woman is sitting there so sadly. Before we have time to reply he says " Perhaps her husband has been killed in the war ". J. adds " Or perhaps her children are always playing funny tricks like Max and Moritz ".

J. is much more inclined than T. to assert himself as far as other people are concerned. T. will permit the same fairy-tale to be told and retold, but J. will not endure it.[1] When adults, perhaps the parents, are speaking among themselves, T. listens and waits for a lull in the conversation before stating his questions and desires, but J. demands to be heard at once and simply will not hear of being put off. If J. is talking to M. or F. he insists that they shall look at him whilst talking, and if they do not do so he seizes their head and turns it towards himself. J. is more belligerent than T. If T. feels himself injured he tends to withdraw into himself and rejects any consolation proffered (16), whereas J. in similar circumstances would launch an attack. If J. feels that his rights have been encroached upon, he begins to brood over plans for revenge (50). He wants to snatch away from the postman the letter to which he thinks he has a claim (64). He thinks out a whole series of

---

[1] Katz, R., " Beobachtungen an Kindern beim Märchenerzählen," *Zeitschr. angew. Psychol.*, vol. 28, 1926.

acts of violence against the whites, who, according to what
he has been told, organized the slave-trade with negroes
in America (74). He threatens to attack the woman who will
not let him have a salamander (127) and does likewise when
he is warned that he is in danger of not getting any of the
things his father has received as birthday presents (130).
J's imaginative play too bears witness to a belligerent spirit
quite lacking in T. When the children in their game have
turned themselves into elves, T. delights the others by his
gymnastics, whereas J. occupies himself chopping down
trees (70). In his dream, real or fictitious (71) J. makes the
thunder take a part. And when T. has complained that a
boy from the kindergarten has thrown sand at him J. is at
once ready with plans for self-help by reprisals (88).

It might perhaps be concluded from these last examples
that T. is less vivacious than J., but that would not give
a true representation of the state of affairs. They are both
lively fellows, but they display it in differing forms and even
on different occasions. In a joyful greeting of his parents,
or in delight at some toy, T. can express the same happy
abandon as J. does in defending his precious titbits and
dainties or in playing with a rabbit. It cannot be said that
the little offences and misdeeds of the two boys differ to
any degree from each other as regards quantity and quality,
and this is probably connected with the fact that misdeeds
are fundamentally governed by temperament.

As is to be expected the differences in the characters of
the children are also revealed in their desires and ideal
future occupations. In an urge for independence J. wishes
for a motor-cycle for himself (3), whilst T. only hopes that
his father will get a car some time, so that he can be taken
too. For a long time J. clung to his choice of sea-captain
as his future occupation. It is in accordance with his urge
for activity and recognition that he is a leader even as a child.
As a parallel to this we may recall that T. had about the
same time the idea of becoming a diver when he grew up.
His object in choosing this occupation was so that he could

observe the marine creatures actually in the water ; that is, the tendency to contemplativeness is here present in contrast to J's activity. As far as the other occupations are concerned, about which the children spoke on occasion, this contrast is not so clearly marked. J's greater tendency to leadership and desire for recognition, which were already present in themselves, were probably fostered by the fact that, as the younger brother, J. was forced more strongly into the attitude of manly protest. The conversations afford numerous examples of this, and we have referred to each individually in the discussions. But the fact that he, as the younger brother, feels pushed into the background occasionally, did not call into being these characteristics. It only caused them to develop to a greater degree than would have been the case had J. been the elder brother.

T's greater tendency to direct his thought inwards probably explains to some extent why he adopts an entirely different attitude towards what he understands as the conception of death than does his brother. He expresses a fear of death very early (33) ; he seems to display a certain reluctance to discuss the death of people with whom he is on intimate terms. On the other hand J. very frequently speaks about the death of others, even about the death of his parents. So perhaps it is not quite accidental that he wants to hear the song about the " burnt " boy—he really thinks it deals with a boy in such a situation. T's habit of directing his thoughts inwards is also revealed in his tendency to self-criticism (55), which reaches an extent never attained even subsequently by J. This self-critical attitude causes T. to refuse a second bag of sweets to celebrate the official beginning of school-life, because, as he says, he has already had one bag (102).

Although both children had a very good sense of humour —we believe better than the average child of their age— yet they displayed it in quite different forms, J's being more robust and T's more intimate. J. is always ready to play the fool and is also delighted if others will do so.

It was not to be expected that all the essential characteristics of the children would be revealed in our conversations. The environmental conditions in the family circle are too uniform to allow of that. But if the social field of force changes, then peculiarities of character hitherto latent are manifested. For instance we had not expected T. to be ambitious, and yet this characteristic appeared when he began to mix in class with school children of about his own age, and had the opportunity of comparing his own performances with those of other children (60). As long as T. was playing only with his younger brother, the adequate social stimulus for bringing out the corresponding impulse was lacking. He was superior to J. in all his performances, so there was no question of any ambition being aroused. The comparison of their own performances with those of adults, causes the children to create an ideal that they would like to grow up to be like their father, but for the present the comparison does not act as a very great stimulus because the gulf between the performances is too wide. Even if the child did not grow up within the family circle and came into closer contact with the stream of the world, many natural attributes of character would still remain dormant in consequence of his generally undeveloped state. These natural attributes are essential elements of a great physical and intellectual maturity, as may be seen if we consider for instance the later types of reaction in the sexual-erotic sphere. As far as other attributes of character are concerned, we may say that they are shown at a very early date in the dynamic form to be in keeping with the childish state. We are sure, for example, that J. will strive for leadership in later life too, and will attempt to assert himself in face of social opposition, just as on the other hand we expect that T., being of a gentler disposition, will be more inclined to try to help his fellow-men. Further observation will of course reveal whether these expectations are fulfilled.[1]

---

[1] On this subject Stern remarks quite correctly (Stern, p. 403), " The individual differences of children with reference to the dynamics of striving

T. never showed the slightest jealousy of his younger brother, but on the contrary he played his part in mothering him. But jealousy was obviously aroused in him when M. began to extend her attention to other children at the opening of the kindergarten. Some of the notes from our diary on this subject are worth communicating. As soon as the parents came to enroll their children at the kindergarten, T. became excited. On the first day when three strange children were going with T. and J. to the playground, T. hit the intruders, took the toys away from them (it was of course a mistake to permit the strange children to have unrestricted use of the toys belonging to T. and J.), knocked down their sand castles and poured sand on them. The next afternoon T. said to M. with tears in his eyes " You ought not to have a kindergarten ". The following day he went to the garden gate early in the morning before the children arrived, held the gate closed and said, " No children shall come, they are thieves, they steal our things." And in the afternoon of the same day the following conversation took place : T. : " I want to earn a lot of money so that you don't need to have a kindergarten." M. : " I don't have the kindergarten in order to earn money, but because I like to have it ". T. : " Why do you like it ? " M : " The children might be run over by motorcars in the street, but if they are with us nothing will happen to them."

After many relapses into his hostile attitude, caused by jealousy (for instance one Sunday, when it was mentioned that the children were not coming, T. remarked : " That's

are very important. And as we are here not dealing with the content, but with the form of difference, they will usually not undergo much change even through the experiences of later life ; they are therefore important for prognosis."—E. Köhler in respect of her " Ann " decided for a development along the lines of Spranger's theoretical man (Köhler, p. 235). Perhaps, however, we are going too far in venturing on a prognostication so early. Indeed any arrangement into types of personality seems questionable when the method of division is based on observations made by adults. Anyone who has no such scruples could regard T. as an introvert and J. as an extrovert type in Jung's sense. C. G. Jung, *Psychologische Typen.*, Zuerich-Leipzig-Stuttgart, 1925.

good, then the cheeky thieves can't come ") T. got accustomed to the coming of the children, and indeed began to like them as playmates. This is shown by the following conversation, which took place about eight weeks after the opening of the kindergarten. T. : " You ought to have more children in your kindergarten." M. : " Why, aren't there enough children there ? " T. : " No, it would be much better to have more children." T. not only allowed the other children to be near him, but he also took care of the smaller ones and was sorry whenever the removal of parents, etc., caused one of the children to leave the kindergarten. The previous spontaneous passionate jealousy entirely disappeared in face of the discovery that his mother's love and devotion to him and his brother were just as great as before, and that the strange children had not caused any difference to this love. This experience was most beneficial to him and made him more mature.

Material collected in the meantime, in conversations and other notes in our diaries, gives an insight into further characterologically important traits in both children. But we must resist the temptation to include this material in view of our remarks in the preface about the extent of time to be covered here.

2. The World of the Child in Content and Form

(a) *The objects of the child's world*

When the folk psychologist describes to us the world of a South-Sea islander or of a South American Indian he is not thinking of the world which the primitive man experiences through his senses, for the primitive sense-organization is scarcely worthy even of passing interest, coinciding as it does almost completely with our own. What the folk psychologist does aim at, is to discover that world dominated by hopes, endeavours, wishes, traditional commands and restrictions, the world as constructed by the savage, which being so totally different from the processes of thought of civilized man is so difficult to approach and even more difficult to appreciate. So here too, when we speak of the world of the child we shall direct our attention to the fantastic hopes and fears, magical ideas and forces which saturate reality for the child and which the child sets up for himself internally with such surprisingly pronounced independence of the organization of his senses which he shares with adults.[1] The world of the child, understood in this sense, represents a unity in itself and by no means sets any problems for the child. It possesses a continuity for which the adult might envy the child.[2] Of this world we may say : " The more primitive stage is not determined by the subtraction of individual characteristics but every stage, however primitive, is a relatively complete organic whole, living its own life." (*Werner*, p. 7.)

[1] The uniformity of sense-organization in children and adults can of course remain concealed even in the simplest experiments in the laboratory. In this connection cf. the illuminating experiments of W. Peters, " Die Entwicklung von Wahrnehmungsleistungen beim Kind," *Zeitschr. Psychol.*, vol. 103, 1927.

[2] Such a view of the world of the child is shared by H. Volkelt in his discussion of the progress of experimental child psychology. *Congress Report*, Jena, 1926.

The world of the child includes first of all what he perceives of its physical surroundings, what he notices, judges, uses and makes into objects to be striven for. This configuration of the surroundings is quite different in a young child from that of the adult. This phrase " of the " must be allowed to stand for the moment, although as is well known in this case too, the aspects of the surroundings with different attitudes and interests, differ from individual to individual. To the child many things do not appear to be present at all, others are overstressed. Articles of furniture which cannot be used for gymnastic exercises, or houses in which no acquaintances live, do not exist at all in the child's consciousness, whereas toys, animate or inanimate can so attract him that the pangs of hunger and extreme tiredness are forgotten. The selective principles dormant in the child, which determine the structure of his world tempt us to speak almost in terms of a different environment for the child, just as Uexküll has done with reference to the various surroundings of various organized animals.[1] What animate and inanimate things exist therefore in the surroundings of the two children under investigation here ? We have not followed up this question systematically, as has been done so often before in the analysis of the stock of ideas in children, e.g. of children starting school, in order to discover what could be presumed as known indeed in their course of education. We have never asked the children if they knew this or that. But nevertheless it is permissible to give a symptomatic meaning to all complexes mentioned in the conversations. What is in a child's heart will certainly overflow through its mouth. It is a much stronger proof of the interest any subject has aroused, if the child begins to talk about it spontaneously, than if the account is only to be obtained by questioning. It is true that the conversations do not give information about all the subjects the child is concerned with inwardly, but the most important categories of these do nevertheless appear, and we can

[1] J. v. Uexküll, *Umwelt und Innenwelt der Tiere*, Berlin, 1909.

testify from a comparison with the numerous dialogues not included, that no essentially new themes occur there.

It is fitting to begin here with the living creatures which populate the world of the child. We shall have occasion to discuss the people of this environment in the section on social-psychological factors, and so we will first of all enumerate the animals with which the children became acquainted either personally in the street, in the Zoo and circus, or in pictures, or finally through stories and conversations. Dogs probably take preference over all other animals. There appear also in the conversations : elephant, wild boar, lion, stag, crocodile, mouse, snail, flea, monkey, salamander, parrot, pigeon, hare, and cockchafer. But the number of animals known to the children and occasionally talked about, far exceeds this list, and includes dozens of animals of the most varied types. The children regarded it as a special favour when they were allowed to look at the illustrations in Brehm, a copy of which was to be found in their father's library. The best-known animals illustrated in this classical animal-book soon became familiar to them. We have already mentioned above the differentiation of character under the influence of intercourse with animals ; even if we disregard for the moment the individual psychological element, there still remains the question of what makes the animal so attractive to children in general. Firstly : every animal arouses pleasure in the child, as a living being, for everything living is much nearer and much more amusing to him than dead things. The child has to some degree a naïve morphological pleasure in animals ; they are enjoyed for the many-sidedness of their forms ; their movements, their games, and when they have young, in their behaviour towards the latter. Under the powerful influence of the extremely anthropomorphistic method of presentation in fairy-tales and other stories, the child ascribes to all animals a human, i.e. his own, mental life. Could there be any more grateful objects for childish fancy than imagining what the squirrel does in his nest on the tree, what the fox does in his lair and how he steals the fowls ? What possibilities are opened up to their play of thoughts by the meetings which one can let animals have one with another. What happens when the lion and the tiger come to grips, or when either of these fights the elephant ? Who is the victor when the eagle attacks the lion, that is, when a flying creature attacks one which is bound to the earth. The child never tires of imagining and thinking out such conflicts. Man is put opposite to animals in the chase. How were the wildest animals captured, those well able to defend themselves, which are to be admired at the Zoo or in the circus ? A minute description of the methods of capturing wild animals in pits is demanded. We have here probably the earliest beginnings of the robber-romantic and love of adventure of older boys. What we have mentioned about the relations towards animals most probably would apply to all boys. It would be interesting to discover what is the position of girls in this matter. Do they treat animals in the same way in their imagination ? Have girls to any extent the same love for animals as we have demonstrated in our boys ? Does a girl's interest only extend perhaps to categories of tamer animals ? In direct connection with the interest in hunting animals is the interest in weapons, such as rifles and cannons.

It might almost be said, that the child's interest in the life of an animal increases in proportion to the strangeness of the animal. The exotic animals which are only known from illustrations or even from literary descriptions attract the child's attention more than the animals of their immediate surroundings. Similarly the child never tires of the joy afforded him by descriptions of strange races of people. The fact that in the conversation negroes are most frequently mentioned is because these people are for the child " the " representatives of strange races. Why is this so ? It is equally as correct to say because the negro impresses the child most with the colour of his skin, which contrasts so strangely with the child's own, as it is to say because negroes appear most often in fairy-tales and other stories as the representatives of foreign races. For they would not appear in fairy-tales which are written for children, unless they were demanded by childish literary taste on account of their popularity. The ethnological interest of the child does not go very deep. The child does indeed listen to stories about the life of negroes, their dress, habits and hunting customs with the greatest attention, but just as he humanizes animals so he europeanizes the negroes; that is, at bottom negroes are regarded as white people painted black, who have adopted such comical and strange habits of life. In addition to negroes there occur in the conversations also Chinese, Eskimos, and among European nations Spaniards, as people giving a strange and foreign impression. We believe we are not mistaken in assuming that the dwarfs who appear in innumerable conversations are understood as a kind of people. The child gets to know the dwarfs as friendly folk and is extremely fond of them.

From childish ethnology it is an obvious step to childish geography. It is not surprising that the home principle is here predominant. Rostock, and places both inside and outside the town, such as the Devil's Pool and Barnstorf, are frequently mentioned. From occasional visits the children know also the Baltic resort Warnemünde and Gehlsdorf, which lies across the River Warnow and which is popular because it is reached by ferry. Because of this the conception " island " is acquired, as it happens not quite correctly in this case. The position of these places in relation to Rostock is clear to the children in the sense that they know how to get to them. That applies also to Denmark and Copenhagen, which, as they know from their own experience, is reached by a huge and extremely interesting ferry-boat. What else do the children know about the world ? On their globe there are also the towns of Cassel and Berlin, as places to which they have been themselves, but better known as the places where relatives live, and whence presents come on birthdays. And finally Göttingen, the town which the

R

parents have told them about in stories of their student-days. The two boys have an emotional rather than scientific geography. Naturally they have no knowledge at all about the true situation of these towns in relation to Rostock. They know that they belong to Germany and compare this country, characterized by the fact that German is spoken there, with other countries, amongst which Russia, France, and Switzerland chiefly occur. Africa and America are the most frequently mentioned extra-European places. All that is known about them is that a long journey by ship is necessary in order to reach them. For some time there was a strong preference, at least in T's case, for the Canary Islands, because his beloved *Robinson Crusoe* had had his adventures there. The children have heard that the earth is round and that it turns, but we have justifiable doubts as to whether they had any accurate idea of the connection between the countries and parts of the world and the whole globe. The contrast between land and water of course influences the geographical ideas of boys living near the sea-coast to a quite different degree from that of children living inland, and so for our children the idea of crossing on the ice to a place usually separated by a stretch of open sea could assume most lively colours.[1]

Mention of *Robinson Crusoe* leads us naturally to speak about the people in mental contact with the child through stories, fairy-tales and various conversations. Amongst the numerous personages who populate the child's inner world, the only serious competitor to *Robinson Crusoe*, and even then only for a short time, was the hero of Scharrelmann's *Berni*. Other characters we may mention are the people in the fairy-tales of Grimm and Hans Andersen : Emperors, Kings, Princes, Princesses and the representatives of the misera plebs. All these people are known only as types, not as clear-cut individual personalities. The same applies

---

[1] The world of peoples whose existence is determined by a life on the sea-coast is described in a valuable little work by E. Reche, *Tangaloa*, Munich and Berlin, 1926.

to groups of people such as the Vikings or other pirates who arouse the interest and admiration of the childish heart by their bold adventurous deeds. Soldiers, as strong, good-humoured fellows are always in favour with boys. They are perhaps a little overshadowed by the fire-brigade when it flashes through the streets with its hoses, to the accompaniment of a clanging bell and the roar of the engine. The present-day policeman enjoyed a much greater popularity with our children than was general years ago.

Workmen who came into the house played a far more important part in the childish world than might be assumed from the conversations. The child is attracted by everything the workman does with his tools. When a workman is in the house the children never leave his side, but in their thoughts too they show interest in manual workers and their jobs, as for instance the joiner, glazier, upholsterer, cobbler, and chimney sweep. The doctor will not be offended if we mention him in this connection also. The children have the greatest confidence in him ; indeed it is more than a parable to say that the child's attitude to the doctor is like that of the savage to the medicine-man. If a doctor has prescribed any treatment, the children take it for granted that he will be obeyed to the letter.

Of Bible-stories the children have learned up to the present Adam and Eve, and David and Goliath ; as the place of the happenings in the Bible they understand Paradise and Palestine. For a long time Goliath was the hero of their childish imagination.

For the sake of completeness we may also mention as people who occur in the conversations, the organ grinder, the porter, and thieves.

Interest in inventions, as for instance in Stephenson, is connected with the conversations about technical discoveries. The children in their own way take a most lively interest in all things technical, for instance in motor cars, motor cycles, railways, post office arrangements, and ships of all kinds, and especially the lifeboat which offers promise of adventure to them. It is quite impossible to discuss individually all the technical things which are mentioned by the children. We believe that quite a different state of affairs exists in this connection among girls, who would not reveal a spontaneous interest in such technical specialities of railway transport as cattle-trucks, milk conveyors, tip-wagons, plate-laying and so on.

With our last remark we have touched on the question of the attitude the child adopts towards the inanimate objects of his environment. Even though the remarks in this second section of our work are not exclusively based on the conversations, but seek to include material from our diaries, yet this additional material must only be used to amplify subjects touched upon in the original conversations, or otherwise we should be embarking on an endless discussion. That applies particularly to this question of the order of importance of inanimate objects in the world of our children, the question with which we will now deal in more detail. It must be remembered that by far the majority of the conversations are not governed and bound by situation, but that they are free conversations. The consequence of this is that they contain relatively little mention of those things in which the child is interested. It must be remembered that the child approaches almost every object with the question " What can I do with this ? " In face of this, the pure impulse for understanding takes second place, just as it does in primitive man. " What can I do with it ? " This question divides the objects with which the child comes into contact into the two main groups of eatables (or perhaps, more correctly, things palatable to the child) and unpalatable things. J., who almost to the present time had the habit of putting anything handy into his mouth, carries out this dividing process directly with his tongue, whilst T. performs it optically. With regard to the unpalatable objects, the child's attitude towards them is decided by the question as to whether he can play on or with them. It is only necessary to extend the conception of play to the sphere of the activity of the imagination in order to get a criterion which actually seems sufficient for assigning all objects, according to their value, to a place in the child's world. The child himself cannot play with a real motor car, motor cycle or lifeboat, but these things can become playthings in his imagination, and therefore assume a high rank amongst the objects of his world.

As far as the ranking of palatable things is concerned we have discussed several points previously in connection with the question of appetite. In their daily life there is more mention of sweetmeats, such as chocolate and bonbons, than one would be led to assume from the comparative rarity with which they are mentioned in the conversations. It must in addition be mentioned that the desire for these things altered very considerably in both children as time went on, and that at certain points of time the appetite for them can greatly change, obviously in close relation to internal and external factors (mood, degree to which demands have been satisfied, time of day and of the year, kind of food already eaten, etc). Strangely enough, if one goes the right way about it, cod-liver oil can also be suggested to the children as a dainty. It appears certain to us that it would not be very difficult to draw up quite a definite table showing the order of preference of dainties and all other food eaten by the children, assuming that external circumstances were kept constant at a given time.[1] Concerning the games of our children and their toys, we may perhaps be allowed to refer to the full discussion of the ways in which children occupy themselves, based on observation of our own children, in a chapter in our book *Die Erziehung im vorschulpflichtigen Alter* (*Education in the pre-school age*). There will be found the observation, always made on such occasions, that the value of a toy for a child

---

[1] D. Katz, "Psychologische Probleme des Hungers und Appetits, insbesondere beim Kinde," *Zeitschrift für Kinderforschung*, 34, 1928.— D. Katz and A. Toll, "Die Messung von Charakter und Begabungsunterschieden bei Tieren," *Zeitschr. f. Psychol.*, vol. 93, 1923, p. 293.

depends least of all on the price charged in the shop. It is not the elaborate costly machine which is always the most coveted toy, but the one with which one can do most. That of course does not exclude ready-made toys from being valued. So the toy-department of a big store is a real children's paradise, and a visit is sufficient to send a child into the seventh heaven of delight. In the conversations balloons are also mentioned : they are attractive both for their colour and shape and for their unusual behaviour. Toys and other means of occupation are subject to fashion ; the child gets tired of them occasionally and after a time returns to them with interest. The money mentioned in the conversations gets its value from the play function attached to it, and not as a means of purchase.

In T. there are the obvious beginnings of a theoretical comprehension of the objects of his environment. This is revealed for instance when he speaks of the nature of light, but the rational consideration of things is only completely triumphant when the child begins to attend school and gets to know the idea of work from first hand experience. In the pre-school age almost all considerations about the surrounding objects start from a practical occupation with them. But this region is left behind with the questions about the origin of living beings and inanimate objects, about death and immortality and also about God. It will cause no misunderstanding if we deal with these questions in the next section, under the title " Metaphysics of the child's world ".

(b) Metaphysics of the child's world

As we have frequently shown, we endeavoured never to burden the children with metaphysical questions touching the religious sphere. But we could not prevent the servants from mentioning such questions to the children, and in a form connected with some definite religious creed. Thus these questions lack clarity to a certain extent.

It appears very questionable to us whether children at this age, with no external stimulus, would ever go so far as to raise, even in the most primitive form, questions about metaphysical problems dealing with God, death, and immortality. But it is certain that they do pursue these questions once the adult has drawn their attention to them ; indeed many conversations betray a little of the absorbed interest which usually only adults devote to these questions. Observation of our children has confirmed the frequently noticed tendency of children to make God into a human being, or even to interpret him as an animal.

In line with all his previous experience the child can only understand the living activities ascribed to God in connection with an organism possessing a body : he cannot comprehend the allegorical sense of all the statements about this subject. In (20) T. asks straight out, " Is God a human being ? " And the same question is repeated by J. in (28), although here the existence of God is immediately disputed, because he cannot be seen. In (32) T. propounds the alternatives that God is either a human being or a bird. The choice of a bird probably arose from the connection of bird and sky or perhaps also from the feeling of a bird's greater mobility.[1] When J. asks whether the Jews existed before God he is acting under the influence of only partially understood information received from Elli, but his reason is drawing upon its own resources when he (53) asks if God was born.[2] For if he understands God to be a human being he is perfectly justified in inquiring about his birth. T. is informed that God is immortal and he deduces quite

[1] A. and K. Busemann in their article, " The Psychology of the Child's Religion," point out the almost unbelievable anthropomorphism in the idea of God observed even in still older children. *Blätter für die Fortbildung des Lehrers und der Lehrerin*, vol. 7, p. 455 et seq.—We mentioned (p. 93) that the young Gottfried Keller regarded God as a bird, namely as the gilded weathercock on a church spire. A little later he connects Him with a splendid tiger, seen in a picture, so that God is to a certain extent a mixture of bird and tiger.

[2] Günther Stern asked his father whether God made himself (Stern, p. 359).

rationally from this that human beings must also be immortal (53). If these questions are once broached the child follows them up and may feel hurt if the adult postpones the requested information by promising to tell him at some later date. But the child's interest is not always equally lively ; for unknown reasons he drops a question and does not take it up again for a considerable time. It is rather improbable that the child would, of his own accord, assume hell to be a place of torment and punishment after death, but if the idea is suggested to him by an adult then it is quite easy to understand that he should feel the desire not to be sent to this place of suffering (99).

The child expresses quite spontaneously the need for information about the origin of a human being (more rarely about his destination), of other animate creatures and of numerous inanimate objects. To the many earlier " Why " questions we now find added the " Whence " and " Whither " questions. Both the " whence " and the " whither ", as we shall soon see, can take on a quite different meaning, but before we go into these differences we must make a more general observation. If the child asks at all about the origin and end of the things in his world, he must already have some mental scheme of this origin and end. The psychological situation implied in the foregoing statement cannot be evaded by merely saying, that the child hears adults speak about the origin and end of things and is just imitating them. That would be a very superficial view of the problem and one which certainly does not coincide with the nature of the process. No, the child works with a systematized anticipation, with a blank formula of the genesis of things which can be filled up in very different ways (Selz). *One* method of filling up the form is known from his own experience, that is the method of *making* for the origin and *destroying* for the end, but experience seems to show him at once that this method does not meet the requirements of the situation. In this intellectual emergency the adult must help him, must correct his experimental beginnings, or inform him of different ways of approaching the subject.

The origin of a human being—to begin with—is inquired about in a two-fold sense : Where does the individual human being come from, and where do human beings in general come from ? The question about the origin of children and about their own origin is very often asked, sometimes spontaneously, sometimes brought up by a situation which induces the question, as for instance if articles of clothing for a new-born baby are seen (67), or if a friend or relative has had an increase in the family. We have stated above that we gave the children information about the natural origin of human beings in a psychologically comprehensible way,[1] but we see that a child will accept quite a different explanation, from its credulous acceptance of the stork fairy-tale, which is even yet preferred by most parents, to an explanation which would be both comprehensible to the child and at the same time true. That this " enlightenment " has by no means the sensational effect which so many parents believe, and which causes them to shirk giving it, is proved by many of our experiences, such as when J. one day expressed the opinion that human beings grew on trees (106). He had therefore temporarily quite forgotten what his parents had told him about the origin of human beings. We had said nothing to the children about procreation ; at present they know only that it is always married people who have children. Later on the children will have to be told the necessary facts in a correspondingly simple and psychologically true way ; but at a time when they do not even know the fundamental difference between the sexes at birth (101) even the most simple statement about procreation would be certainly premature. T. begins spontaneously to talk about the birth of twins, and has his own special ideas on the subject (19).

The children know from their own observation of plants, animals, and lastly human beings, that a larger being can

---

[1] The pedagogical basis is given in Katz, *Erziehung*.

develop from a smaller one by the process of growth. The growth of human beings is most forcibly impressed on them by the fact that experience shows them that their clothes become too small for them in course of time. They have also been shown some of their own baby-clothes and go into raptures at their doll-like dimensions. They are only too willing to hear about the time when they were as small as that. Is this due to the delight in minute things, or is there an admixture of pride at now being so much bigger ? [1]

The child's question about the " whence " of human beings has also a phylogenetic as well as an ontogenetic sense. The child sees himself placed in the line of parents, and grandparents, which he can follow. On the other hand he learns about Adam and Eve and about their children and children's children (20). Probably he has a presentiment of the connection between the two fragments of the whole series of generations, without, however, possessing the correct scientific ideas which alone would make the series a connected whole. Between the existence of human beings and that of animals no connection is suspected, whilst many questions seem to touch on the idea of descent, in so far as it is only concerned with animals.

The child also raises the " whence " question in another sense, with reference to dwarfs and giants. How can one become a giant, why does one remain so small ? The special case needs a special explanation. Explanations of the most varied value are accepted by the child as logical. Why did Goliath become a giant ? The child is equally satisfied with the answer that Goliath came from the giant's town, or that his mother always gave him so much to eat, or that he always washed in cold water.

There is perhaps a trace of the theory of descent in T's question, whether animals existed before human beings (32). He also asks generally which animals existed formerly (30), and how elephants and horses developed. But he seems

[1] Compare in this connection A. Busemann, " Die Freude der Kinder am besonders Grossen und Kleinen," *Zeitschr. angew. Psychol.*, vol. 24, 1924.

rather to have a new creation in mind, in so far as he is thinking at all about the appearance of new types of animals. Perhaps at first God created everything different, so that the animals, even snakes, could talk. It seems clear to both children that a large animal cannot develop from a small one (for instance an elephant from a flea), yet J. thinks it possible for flowers to become trees by growing. J's question about the origin of meat and straw, in the conversation about the origin of animals, shows that he uses this category of origin in a far wider sense than does T. at the same time. For J., organic development is not yet distinct from mechanical manufacture. J. mingles as identical questions about the origin of guns, trees, flowers, and tomatoes (24). Again, information which is logically of quite varied value is capable of satisfying the child, as for instance, in the question about the origin of guns, the answers that they are made in factories or that they are bought in shops. T's assumption that towns must have been empty at first, and then inhabited by people, is a good mistake. The children's geological suppositions—there must have been a lake where Rostock now lies—have been developed by thinking about information learned in conversation.

It would probably be easy to carry out numerous illuminating investigations into parallelism in the ideas of children and primitive man with reference to the origin of things. But when we come to consider the problem of the end of things, the death of human beings and animals, we find only a scanty material in child psychology to put forward against the amazingly extensive mass of evidence yielded by ethnology. We tried in every way to keep from our children the idea of the death of people, and we believe that a similar reticence, common to most parents in dealing with this subject, has had an unfavourable influence on the accumulation of material which would help us towards an understanding of the child's attitude towards death. An additional factor is, as Stern remarks, that the idea of death can scarcely be comprehended by the child at all. It is true that in fairy-tales there is a great deal—indeed too much—about striking dead, burning to death, hanging, and other methods of causing the transition from life to death, but the child does not comprehend what really lies behind it. For the child, death in fairy-tales probably means nothing more than " not playing any longer ", the withdrawal of the person concerned. Our children also spoke quite often about murder and shooting in the shallow sense just mentioned, but a presentiment of the tragedy behind death is only to be seen in one conversation with T. (33). He asks if everything living comes to an end, and in conjunction he expresses the desire to live, if not for ever, at least longer than all other people. From his attitude and tone of voice, rather than from the actual formulation of the words, it was clear that the child had been touched by the seriousness of the problem of death. Although psychoanalysts record numerous cases where boys are said to have desired the death of their father, whom they considered as a rival, we are inclined to assume that even in these cases—supposing that the psychoanalyst has correctly interpreted the child's behaviour—the wish expressed was that the father should stop playing the game and disappear, rather than that he should be completely destroyed.[1]

As we have demonstrated elsewhere [2] we tried for a long time to keep from the children the idea that the meat eaten at table originated from animals which had been killed. Subsequent experience showed us that the pedagogic scruples, which had led us to this conduct, were not justified to the extent we thought. The children had not the slightest disinclination to eat the poultry which they had seen lying whole in the kitchen in the form of an unplucked chicken,

---

[1] Sully reports the case of a little girl 3½ years old, who did not want to die. She begged her mother to place a large stone on her head, in order to prevent her from growing and so from getting older. T. Sully, Leipzig, 1904.

[2] Katz, *Erziehung*.

and whose preparation they would follow—in so far as they were allowed—with the greatest interest. They had—and this applies also to T.—not the slightest fear of touching dead animals and of playing with them. Once a tom-tit got into the house and before we could prevent it, killed itself by flying against the window, but even this sudden transition from life to death did not have the depressing effect which we had expected, and which indeed we ourselves felt at the event. Instead the children picked up the dead bird, fully expecting that they would be able to make it move again. They simply did not grasp the fact that all was over with the little creature. There can be no pessimism in a world where death has no power over the mind, and indeed the essence of an optimistic outlook on life can never be studied in greater concentration than in children of this age.

(c) *The wish world of the child*

However much we try as adults to keep our view of the world free from wishes and hopes, fears and anxieties, our outlook on life will always be influenced in quite a legitimate way, in its coarser and finer traits, by these subjective moments. And where can the influence of one's outlook on life on one's theoretical comprehension be absolutely excluded ? The ideals of the adult are crystallized out from his " wish pictures," which by no means rarely can be traced back to the earliest years of childhood. If they are considered critically they can to some extent be separated from raw reality. But at the age of our children the world which is being built up internally is still completely and inextricably mingled with their wishes and hopes. People believe what they wish. This statement applies without any limitations to the child, and the extent to which the child's belief determines the shape of his world, can be clearly seen from the foregoing conversations. It may perhaps be doubtful whether the child speaks more of the past or of the future at the age in question, but it is quite certain that his feelings are much more devoted to coming things.

The child refers to the future innumerable times with the phrase " when I grow up ". The frequency of this phrase alone, quite independent of any special statements about the future, shows what an attraction it has for him. What is the future to bring to a boy ? His ideal is size and strength, which for him are almost synonymous. Probably every healthy boy has this heroic ideal. *Adler* is therefore unquestionable right on this point, but it seems to us unnecessary to assume, as he does, that it is always connected with a sense of one's own inferiority and incapacity. This latter may perhaps be true of J. within certain limits. As already mentioned, J. must occasionally experience his own inferior capacities in comparison with his elder brother, but this is not true of T., who can have only the positive wish to be big and powerful and strong in the future. This wish is usually expressed in the more concrete form " to grow up like Papa ". J. probably feels his distance behind T. rather painfully, but we do not suppose that this applies to T's relation to his father. There are two reasons for this ; the distance between T. and father is too great for the necessary comparison to be made (comparisons are always made with people of similar capacities, not with those quite dissimilar) and secondly, T. loves his father too much for any feelings of inferiority and envy to have their starting-point in the object of his affection. T. wants to look like his father and protests with mournful looks when acquaintances, all unsuspectingly, deny that there is any resemblance between him and his father. It is perhaps not quite so accidental a choice of words as it appears, when J. does not express the wish to be like Papa, but instead to be Papa (3), that is, he claims the father's position and influence immediately for himself. We believe that the interest in Goliath, expressed in so many conversations, is coloured by the desire to become like this giant whom they idolize, and that this interest cannot be set parallel to the purely platonic interest in dwarfs as the counterpart of giants. No child expresses the wish to be always a dwarf in the future, however much his childish imagination adores the lovable little creatures. Indeed it is expressly laid down as a hygienic necessity that the children must have plenty of fresh air, so that they may not remain as small as a certain gentleman of their acquaintance (121).

The theme of the future profession occupies a good deal of space in the conversations. What are the decisive motives in a child's choice of profession ? Leaving aside all individual differences, which are so revealing as an indication of character, we may say that those professions are chosen where there is plenty of incident, where things happen, and where there is a prospect of meeting with adventures. As a rule the choice of a profession is not adhered to very long, for even the nursery has its fashions so far as choice of profession is concerned. For some almost inexplicable reason one day, a new profession is mentioned, after the old one has been sufficiently enjoyed in imagination and become stale. The following are the most important of the professions chosen by the children in chronological order, but without assigning them in every case to one or other of the children. First sea-captain and porter, then sailor, engine-driver, mail van-driver, waiter, and guard. Then another sea-coast profession occurs, the diver. J. wants to become a teacher, then a poet. Finally he definitely rejects the profession of sea-captain because he cannot swim.

What is rejected is really just as characteristic as what is wished. Naturally the children do not speak as often about the things they detest as they do about the things they like. But where that occurs, the decisive rejection bears witness to the strength of feeling lying behind it. Just as the devil is the counterpart of God in the world, the child, influenced by the construction of most fairy-tales, opposes the favourite characters of the world of his imagination to those he dislikes. For both our children the prototype of all dreaded beings was the witch, who occasionally haunted their dreams also. Of course the witch is not an autonomous creation of childish imagination but rather due to the gratuitous aid of servants in their fairy-tales and stories. But the fact that the witch is endowed with all the children's ideas of wickedness seems to indicate a deep necessity of having at their disposal a personal representative for the negative side of their values also. Fairy-tales introduced the children to other representatives of evil, baseness and spitefulness but none made the same impression as the witch.[1] Is it not possible that we have here the influence of the exact opposite to the mother, who seems to the child the incarnation of goodness to a much higher degree than does the father ?

We mentioned previously the great love the children had for animals. There is really only one exception, the snake, a dislike of which was probably taken over from adults. The children have never yet seen a live snake and so in the imaginative animal-world of the children it can play the part of the evil principle which the witch performs amongst human and similar beings.

Everything that the children have heard about war— that people starved, that many children lost their fathers, that all concerned suffered in some way, produced in them a great loathing of war. This applies particularly to T., in whom the idea of a future war—the parents' discussions of newspaper articles, etc. touch on this question occasionally —arouses violent feeling.

The children have as yet no reflective relation to their own health ; this may be connected with the fact that they have up to the present fortunately escaped illness which would have kept them in bed any length of time. When J. expresses the wish in (91) to be well on his approaching birthday, he is less concerned with the momentary evil, which would be thereby removed, than with the sorry situation which would result if all the children came to celebrate his birthday with him and he could not take part.

---

[1] Many fairy-tales were put before our children in an " adapted " form. Further details in Katz, *Erziehung*.

Birthdays in general, together with other festive days usually made memorable by the invitation of friends of the children, form the most important orientation points for the future. They are therefore ideas connected with joyful feelings which lead to the conquest of a new sphere, here the future. The birthday table, which is " almost " going to break beneath the load of presents (91), affords for a long time in the child's time-perspective an important fixed-point for his deliberations about things lying more distant in time.

Their future attendance at school is much less frequently the subject of the child's thoughts than is the future profession.   This is easily understood from the fact that the child promises himself very little amusement from attendance at school. The wishes expressed by T. (59) with regard to his later attendance at school, do not arise from any personal estimates of value, but have been adopted from understood descriptions given by older friends.

We may once again mention that T., in connection with his estimate of the value of fruit, expresses the hope that he will be able to live in Italy at a later date, whereas J., more indefinite, speaks only of living " in the country ", which probably, from the descriptions he has heard, seems to him the main source of supply of meat.

Concerning the children's wishes about the future form of the family, we may chiefly mention their frequently expressed wish for a little brother, in order to be able to play with him.

(d) Orientation in time

The foregoing remarks lead easily to a general discussion about the orientation of the child in time, for which our conversations supply some material. It must be stated that at the time the preceding conversations ended, even T. had still a remarkably poor orientation in time, without in any way lagging behind the average child of his age.[1]

---

[1] The majority of six-year-olds are not yet clear about the meaning of the words minute, hour, week, and month. Bühler, p. 143.

It is well known that during these early years the child has still very few standards of time to judge by, and those which he has he can only use imperfectly. To a greater extent than the adult the child lives in the present, and is more closely connected with it by the emotional trend of his existence. Long before the child begins, as adults do, to apply periodic happenings and the units of time arising from these to the course of events, he divides these events which are noticed, affectively into the single happenings of each individual day (breakfast, afternoon sleep, evening meal, etc.) or of each year (birthdays, Easter, Christmas, etc.), so that there results a more qualitative division of very irregular structure.

We note from the conversations that the children almost certainly regard the day they have just lived through as a time unit, for it is only in exceptional cases that they include more remote events in their retrospect of the day. It may very well be assumed that for an accurate estimation the same criteria will be applied as occur in the case of adults on similar occasions ; i.e. clearness and richness of ideas, exclusiveness, promptness, and persistence of reproduction.[1] If in this connection the child makes false localizations in time the confusion is very widespread, and " yesterday " is scarcely to be distinguished from " three days ago " or from " some weeks ago ".

The children again are quite surprisingly uncertain as to the meaning of young and old as applied to human beings. We recall here T's question about his father's age (10), and the conversation (4) where J. thinks it possible that his mother is sewing on a button which had come off father's trousers when he was still a little boy. All people who appear grown-up (i.e. big) to the children, seem to be for them about the same age. At times, however, the fact of being an adult is not determined by qualities which the person possesses in himself, but simply according to whether he has parents

---

[1] G. E. Müller, *Zur Analyse der Gedächtnistätigkeit und des Vorstellungsverlaufes*, part 3, sect. 10, Leipzig, 1913.

still living or not (116). If one still has parents one cannot be grown-up ; it will be recognized to what a degree all these temporal estimates of the child are saturated in qualitative considerations. When J. (127) asks if the spots caused by the plaster will have disappeared by his wedding day, we have evidence both of the boy's lack of knowledge about the age at which people usually marry, and also about the probable time such a spot will last. In every case where the children speak about the professions they intend to adopt later on, their ideas have the quality sign " future " ; these ideas, however, are devoid of any quantitative time-sense. That is true also for the cases where their own future attendance at school is being discussed, although here they are dealing with extents of time which are easier to grasp. After all this we can expect nothing concerning the historical understanding of children. The remote event of general significance, which the children spoke most about, was the war, as they themselves knew, a time before they were born. The fact that Goliath's opponent and their father bore the same name, caused the children to make their father a contemporary of the giant. We find the rudiments of a historical sense in conversation (23), where tradition preserved in books is being discussed. We get a connection made between temporal and geographical things in (79) and (103), where there is revealed a certain understanding of the fact that it can be night at a certain place on the earth whilst it is still day at another. Conversation (48) reveals that the idea of distance connected with ideas of time is still very inaccurate.

We close this discussion with a test-conversation with T., made on 18th February, 1927, that is about four months after the last recorded conversation. F. carried out this test with the express object of discovering the boy's position at this time as regards certain ideas of time.

F. : " How long is a week ? "
T. : " Seven days."
F. : " How long is it still before your birthday ? "

T. : " Three months perhaps, or six."

F. : " Who will have a birthday first, Julius or you ? "

T. : " Julius."

F. : " How long is a year ? "

T. : " Do you mean how many days ? I don't know."

F. : " Is a year long or short ? "

T. : " Long."

F. : " Were you in Copenhagen or Warnemünde last ? "

T. : " Last ? Do you mean when I am dead ? "

F. : " No, I mean, is it longer since you were in Copenhagen or in Warnemünde ? "

T. : " It's longer since Copenhagen."

F. : " How long is a day ? "

T. : " Eleven or twelve hours."

F. : " Do you sleep longer or are you awake longer ? "

T. : " About the same. When the curtains are drawn the night is longer."

F. : " Does Easter or Christmas come first ? "

T. : " Christmas comes first."

F. : " What season is it now ? "

T. : " Winter."

F. : " What season comes then ? "

T. : " First Spring, then Summer, then Winter."

F. : " You've forgotten one. Which season comes before Winter ? "

T. : " Autumn."

Since T. has been attending school his orientation in time has very rapidly made considerable progress.

(e) The Dreams of Children

There are only a few observations available concerning the dreams of children at an early age. We would mention the details Bühler gives on this subject. Just as has been done so frequently with animals, Bühler with the utmost reserve assumes the possibility that children dream, from various expressive movements occurring in sleep.[1] Stern gives some details about dreams as related by the child

[1] Bühler, ch. 6.

himself.[1] The findings about dreams recorded by Carla Raspe were collected from school-children.[2]

As Stern has expressly pointed out, it is necessary to be extremely cautious in considering the statements of young children about their dreams. It seems to us that an important criterion of the reliability of the account, is its spontaneousness, and so far as the content is concerned, the originality of the dream as compared with other imaginary reports given by the child. We believe that for at least some of the dreams mentioned by us, these criteria prove the reliability of the children's statements. This applies for the first dream, mentioned in conversation (34).

T. gave a spontaneous account of it, and its content is quite different from the usual products of the boy's imagination. It seems probable to assume that the dream about the moon falling down and rolling across the street is influenced by the genuine experience of the shooting-star, which the boy mentions in his account immediately after the narration of the dream. From its content we are inclined to count the dream about the black mask from conversation (70) also as genuine, even though the report was only given in reply to his mother's question. From the details given in (65) we think it probable that T. really does know the sensation of hovering from his own previous dreams, and that it is not merely a waking imagination or the adoption of another person's statements. As we have previously stated we cannot bring ourselves to ascribe a sexual motive to this dream of hovering, as is done by many psycho-analysts, but we consider a psychological interpretation is more likely, such as we find for instance in *Vold*.[3] The dream about the black mask may probably be classed as a decided wish-dream, but the same does not apply to the dream about the moon, which reveals a slight attack of fear.

---

[1] Stern, p. 258 et seq.

[2] Carla Rapse, " Untersuchungen über Kinderträume," *Zeitschr. päd. Psychol.*, vol. 25, 1924.

[3] Mourly Vold, *Über den Traum*, Leipzig, i, 1910 ; ii, 1912.

It is possible that when the boy saw the shooting-star, he feared a more serious catastrophe of a similar nature, this time with the moon.

What the younger boy reports does not quite bear the same stamp of truth. It is not absolutely impossible that J. dreamt about an elephant with two legs, but is quite feasible also that he only imagined it. It is scarcely to be doubted that J. had dreams, and his spontaneous statement in the same conversation that he often dreams of nasty things, may be quite accurate. But he does not succeed to the same extent as his brother in gaining possession of his dreams so that he can report them afterwards.

We append here two further dreams about which, according to our diary, T. gave two spontaneous reports. The one is remarkable for the unusual force with which it had its effect in the waking state, the other for a peculiar linguistic achievement taking place in a dream. One morning T. came to his father's bed and without saying a word began to feel his father's wrist. When asked why he was doing this he replied that he had dreamed that he was walking across the market square in Rostock accompanied by his father, when a horse came and bit the father in the place he was now touching. The father showed the boy, who was very distressed, that the hand was quite uninjured, but the boy would not be consoled by this, but instead seized the other arm and examined the wrist with the same thoroughness as he had done the first. Both investigations were performed with such care that they resembled a medical examination, and from this could be judged that the dream experience had been exceptionally powerful. The experience must have had the strength of a powerful hallucination. It would be turning things completely upside down if one were to read into this dream a wish-dream, in which the desire to harm or remove the father has played a part. T. always shows himself touchingly concerned for his father's well-being and becomes perturbed if he thinks he sees him in a dangerous situation. Such a harmless situation, falsely interpreted by T., probably was one of the contributory causes of the dream. The second dream was one in which a remarkable linguistic performance was accomplished. T. told us that he had dreamt about a town inhabited entirely by witches. This town had the name " Zigzag ". T. knew the word zigzag from ordinary conversation ; although it is not often used, it had probably impressed the boy with its unusual sound. The transfer of this word to a mysterious town, whose only inhabitants are witches, seems to us a really excellent performance in a child's dream, for we have no indication that it was suggested to the child either by us or by any other person with whom he came into contact.

We know that both children dream much more frequently than would be assumed from their reports, from the numerous occasions on which they wake with a start. If they are then questioned, they usually reply that they have been dreaming but have forgotten what it was about. For the personal attitude of the child towards his dreams the quite casual question in conversation (45) is noteworthy : Why does one not dream about what one has thought about ? Is it already recognized that the same authority cannot be exerted over the events of dreams as is exerted over the events of the waking mental life ? We shall soon have to discuss the categories of reality in the world of the child, but we may remark at this point that in our experience the boundary between the world of ideas in dreaming and that of the waking life is by no means as fluid as is still represented in many investigations. The only case where we may speak with certainty of the influence of a dream experience being effective in waking consciousness was in T's dream about his father being injured by a horse, and this must be considered an exceptional case. At this age the child is obviously kept from referring these experiences more often to reality in the same way as the adult is, by simply forgetting the more fleeting dream pictures.

(f) The categories of reality in the world of the child and magical thinking in children

We have just rejected the widely-held theory that the reality of the child's dream is effective to a high degree in his waking world. For only a single certain case of belief in the reality of a dream-happening has been discovered by us up to the present. What is the position with regard to the other spheres of reality of the child ? Werner remarks on this subject : " There is actually only a relatively slight differentiation between the child's spheres of reality, whether it is a question of the reality of a dream or of art as opposed to everyday practice (p. 122). . . . Many factors play their part in bringing about the merging of the spheres of reality. . . . The events of the (child's) waking hours may often be shaped by the emotions of fear and desire (p. 122). . . . When the child is playing, is he conscious of the make-believe character of the game, or is he living in this world just as in the world of waking reality ? In my opinion it is quite wrong to ask this question in such a clear-cut form, for it is being asked from the standpoint of the ways of experience of the normal educated adult. It may be demonstrated that a waking reality of this preciseness does not exist at all in the child, and so cannot be brought forward as such as a contrast to the reality of play " (p. 127).

It is advisable to connect with these quotations from Werner, our own observations on the question of the relation of the child's spheres of reality one to another. On the basis of our personal experience we must at once reject the fusing of the reality of dreams and waking life which Werner assumes. Is it that Werner is thinking of an earlier age, or is it because our children were, to a special degree, proof against the intermingling which threatened here ? We prefer to think that other authors have generalized in an unpermissible way about individual experiences which pointed in this direction. We have practically never been able to discover a confusion of those events about which we had only told the children and those which they had themselves experienced.   How do our children behave towards the unreal world of art ?   In this we group together the child's games, first amongst them the important character acting—even when adults take part in it—their behaviour towards plays seen in the theatre, the literary art, chiefly the fairy-tale and pictorial art.

Hetzer made children play definite parts and observed them as they were playing these games.[1]   She comes to the conclusion that in children's games we usually have to deal with make-believe interpretations, and only in rare cases with those taken seriously.   The expressions of emotion manifested during the games were far less vivid than those revealed at corresponding actual events.   From our own innumerable observations, of which naturally only an extremely small number could be utilized in the recorded conversations, we think we are justified in assuming that Hetzer met with so little emotional manifestation in the games, simply because she was observing games started by her own external impulse.   In the character-acting games, which daily grow up spontaneously out of the child himself, the most lively manifestations of emotion are the rule and not the exception.   We agree with Werner's warning against assuming in the child a waking reality of the same preciseness as the adult knows.   Therefore the experiencing of his own personality is not so definite and limited in the child as it is in the adult, and therefore it is much easier for the child to lose himself without restraint in the role he is portraying in a character-play.   At the age with which we are here concerned the child is constantly prepared to transform himself into someone else.   He is always on the alert, ready to jump into any character suggested by the situation, or even to impersonate animals, and to maintain the role

---

[1] Hildegard Hetzer, *Die symbolische Darstellung in der frühen Kindheit*, Wien, 1926.   This work also contains some conversations, recorded word for word, which took place during the play.

with great emotional power. He is father or mother, bride or bridegroom, merchant or sea-captain, he is at an hotel or on a journey. The conversation, manner of speech, movements and behaviour, are all adapted to the part played. It is astonishing how the child's store of experience, which at the best can be but small, is drawn on it order to build up the most varied worlds in these character-plays. For anyone who is not very sure of his own personality as a constant it does not mean so much to give up this personality to the experience of another person, whom he has got to know by some quite casual means. " For the child anything is real which is experienced intensely " (*Stern*, p. 245). Thus the child can experience himself as a horse, tiger, lion or bear, or he can experience other people as such. The bear, into which the mother has turned herself (35) is feared by J. There is no question of J. only pretending to be afraid, he is really very frightened, and even T. has to confess that it felt a little uncanny to him when his mother growled. The mother is mother and bear all in one ; she can transform and re-transform herself at a word. This phenomenological state cannot be brushed aside by merely labelling it the child's " strong suggestibility " or " primitive credulity ", for, apart from the fact that we cannot in general speak of strong suggestibility and primitive credulity in connection with our children, such a course would only mention by name the producing factors, but would leave unmentioned the state itself.[1] It is by no means always necessary that these should be the suggestive effect of an adult personality to make the child believe in a magic transformation into another human or animal personality. The children play tricks on each other, even the younger brother teases the elder, as (109) reveals. The disenchantment takes place just as speedily and painlessly as the reverse

---

[1] In experiments on capacity to express oneself, on being shown a picture (Stern's method) the two children showed themselves quite inaccessible by suggestive questions. On the same occasion they showed an inner freedom which surpassed that of many an uneducated adult.

process. We have clear examples of changes of personality in (56). Quite naïvely J. presupposes the same capacity for illusion in adults as he himself possesses. How often has J. come into the room slightly disguised—perhaps with just a cloth round his head and his face quite uncovered—firmly convinced that he will not be recognized. He is extremely pleased when his parents do not recognize him at all and take him for a tramp or some stranger. Then he unmasks and calls out in tones of mingled triumph and reassurance " Of course it's Julius ". Thus he thinks he will easily be able to deceive the railway official and be taken for a clown if he puts on a little colour (98). Just as striking for the adult as the child's belief in arbitrary changes of personality, is the loss of a person's character, which takes place for the child without the adult being able to see any reason for it. We mention in this respect J's mistake about his mother, made on the excursion (82). In the test-conversation about T's identity, J. did indeed at first offer resistance to the suggestive prompting, but finally his belief began to waver. At times it was only necessary for father to say quite definitely " I am not Papa " in order to confuse the children about his person, whereupon they would turn to their mother and ask whether it really was Papa. Transformation of persons into other persons, or into animals and objects, are of course known to the children from fairy-tales, but this is not their reason for considering these transformations possible in the case of persons of their own surroundings. Rather is the reverse the case : by reason of their mental make-up they consider transformations possible and so they understand similar transformations in fairy-tales. The language in which this mental structure finds expression originates, of course, as the frequent repetition of the word " bewitch " shows, principally from the fairy-tale. We see from the conversations referring to visits to the theatre, that the reality of the theatre is at first not distinguished from that of everyday life.

Although the child so frequently asks questions about the existence of persons, animals, and objects by using the formula " Is there really . . . ? " yet this " really " does not mean only the adult's sphere of reality but is just as likely to refer to the sphere of the fairy-tale, of figurative imitation of stories and of the imagination. The children know that dwarfs really exist in the stone figures in the garden, the illustrations in books and in fairy-tales. They have their existence only in these forms ; therefore it causes a dreadful confusion, when dwarfs dare to force their way as living beings also into the child's world (21). Witches and Santa Claus, angels and devils, and all the other human and animal figures in fairy-tales and stories exist really *in their sphere* ; unless the child were informed, he would not have the slightest appreciation of the fact that these figures are nothing but figments of the imagination, which only exist by permission of the imagination. If the child is told that there are no real devils and witches and is consoled by the information, he does not interpret it as meaning that he will be certain of not meeting devils and witches in the street, but the information takes away the imaginative existence from these terrifying figures. It tells the child in a suggestive form ; you need not be in the least disturbed by them. These figures are therefore exorcized (only) in the world of imagination, and the child is helped by this means. J's questions as to whether there are really musicians and crocodiles (30) or girls on wheels (31), probably refer to the occurrence of these neither in nature nor in imagination—which are by no means clearly distinguished in this case—but seek to obtain information about the things in question and what can be done with them and how they can be utilized in the imagination. This last statement applies chiefly to the younger boy, while T. has already a clearer idea of what can truly be called " really " and what only exists in the imagination. As was to be expected, theatre-illusion persists longest in T's case, but the beginning of his freeing from this is shown, e.g. in places in the theatre-conversation (11) and in (140), where T. makes an attempt to distinguish between the actors and their parts, even though he fails in the effort.

Our diary gives numerous examples of the fact that objects with which the children play are treated as alive in some way by the younger child. We have two instances of this in our conversations. In (1) J. apostrophizes the cookery-book as a rude book, but then withdraws the remark as if he feared he might have offended the book, which he then terms a good book. In (64) J. asks in all seriousness whether the letter rang the bell, and here we are not dealing with a slip of the tongue or poetic licence. Thus the boundaries between realities appear to be removed here—boundaries between animate and inanimate things, which the adult cannot cross.

Animals and people in pictures, and represented plastically, are treated as being alive. Thus J. endeavours to let the dwarfs in the cookery-book see his new sweater ; " they will laugh " (2). The cause of the grief of the woman in Dürer's *Melancholie* is inquired into ; her real existence is never once doubted. An illustrated figure becomes most vivid and alive if it is already known from a previous story, as for instance happens in the case of *Robinson Crusoe*. In J. we find confusion between what he has experienced and what he has most fervently desired.

What are the causes of this confusion of the boundaries between the various realities of the child ? They are to be sought principally in the lack of separation of the child's thinking, feeling, and wishing. The emotional thinking is extremely strong, the rational comprehension of reality frees itself with difficulty from the bonds of feeling and wishing which hold it fast. Emotion is the strongest motive force of the child's mental activities in general and of his thinking in particular, but it is at the same time also the greatest obstacle to a logical manner of thinking. Emotion can cause the child to rise to high performances, as when J., fearing to be separated from his mother, casts about for arguments to prevent it (88), but emotion often leads astray, as for instance when T., fired by the desire to grow, makes a statement on this subject which he cannot substantiate (21). The progress in thinking takes place as a freeing from wishes, hopes and fears. As long as this emancipation is not completed we may speak of a magical thinking rooted in emotions, which is accompanied by an attempt towards an equally emotionally determined (i.e. magic) control of environment in all its varied forms. However much imaginary strength magic thinking induces in a person, yet, considered objectively, it is always a sign of weakness, namely a sign that the technique either of the physical or the psychical world is not viewed with sufficient clarity as to really master it, or—to forego its mastery.

We now turn to the question of magical thinking in the child, a subject which deserves attention both in itself and also because we here meet with the most interesting parallels between the child's thinking and the thinking of primitive man.[1] Some notes on the question of magical thinking are given in the work of C. Raspe mentioned on p. 37, although here the author's main interest was not specifically devoted to this question. Werner has treated the subject of magical thinking in all its development and historical importance in much greater detail, and thus he deals with magical thinking in the psychology of the child, primitive man, and the feeble minded. It may justly be said that the magical way of thinking is not illogical and not prelogical but simply logically different from that of the normal adult. At the same time that the child is still paying tribute to magical thinking in one sphere, he may in another sphere be able to draw conclusions which can only be classified as ingenious. This is not mutually exclusive, since the influence of emotion, and therefore dependence on it, varies in

[1] The most important modern works on the psychology of primitive man, in which the original intimate connection between idea, feeling, and will as a precondition for magic thinking is demonstrated, come from L. Lévy-Brühl, (1) *Les fonctions mentales dans les sociétés inférieures*, 1 Aufl., Paris, 1910 ; (2) *La mentalité primitive*, Paris, 1922.

intensity in various spheres. T. deduces from the agreement of two clocks that they are showing the correct time, but at the same time he allows himself to be terrified by his younger brother's statement that he has changed himself into a dangerous animal (wolf).[1] All our illustrations of the child's credulous acceptance of the transformation to one person into another person or into an animal are to be regarded as the effect of magical thinking. Werner has not investigated in detail the way in which the child's magical thinking, here displayed, is set in action. In so far as it does not take place spontaneously and thus preclude further explanation, the expressively spoken word, in conjunction with an unaccustomed and unusual gesture, reveals itself as very effective. There are, however, also certain subjective moments which must be fulfilled before word and gesture can have their suggestive effect. The child is not always equally receptive and in one mood will reject a suggestion which would be immediately taken up in another mood. Let us recapitulate what we consider to be magical thinking according to the definition just given. In addition to the above-mentioned transformations of human beings into other human beings, and into animals, we may also point to the occasional mistaking of near relatives noticed in J. The most intense experiences from the character-plays should also probably be included here as autistic transformations. The beginning of magical thinking proper by the child may perhaps even be made to coincide with the beginning of the character-plays. Autistic transformations of personality presuppose experience of other personalities to an extent as yet beyond the reach of the young child. As far as our observations up to the present go, it seems that

---

[1] Primitive man also is not inextricably rooted in magical thinking, but his usefulness and adaptability in many technical matters shows that he is able to think logically and to learn from experience. According to Vierkandt (Review of Levy-Suhl, "Neue Wege in der Psychiatrie," *Zeitschr. angew. Psychol.*, vol. 28, 1926) the difference between us and primitive man does not exist on the logical side but on the side of the varying content of the thinking, that is the differences in *Weltanschauung*.

the stricter discipline in thinking which begins when the child begins to attend school, breaks down the child's magical thinking, and indeed is intended to do so, but this magical thinking is quite capable of finding new retreats somewhere in the mind. In fact, is there any educated civilized person who claims to be quite free from the slightest remnant of magical thinking? Whose thinking—even political—is quite uninfluenced by any emotions? In his explanation of magical transformations in children, Werner is quite right in stressing the diffuse and complex character of the child's ego, his indefinite boundaries in his relations to other people, his relatively incomplete strength. It is no contradiction of this to note for instance that each of our children was able to distinguish his own eating utensils, even though they were similar to his brother's, and would refuse the other's. T. intends a magic action when (87) he hopes to be able to order good weather by a letter sent into the sky. Transformations based on word-magic, the model of which is probably to be sought in fairy-tales, are to be seen in those cases where the child turns himself into some animal or other with the formula " I am now. . . . " [1] The influence of medicine is also regarded by the child as magical (95).

From our diaries we append the following further magic actions, which really took place. When we had a boiled fowl at table, T. begged to be allowed to eat the neck, and he added spontaneously: so that he could breathe better. Here we have a very good example of " participation magic ", dealt with at such great length by folk-psychology. About this time T. had complained several times that he found it difficult to breathe. He probably thought the neck was the breathing organ, both in himself and in animals. By incorporating the fowl's neck in himself he now hoped obviously to acquire the bird's capacity for breathing.

[1] W. Krogmann in a work on magical thinking in the child, which contains many good observations, tries to trace this thinking back to " emergency thinking ". This does not seem to us generally permissible. *Zeitschr. f. pädag. Psychologie*, vol. 27, 1926.

The case is especially conclusive since we ourselves had never expressed such ideas in the boy's presence, nor, so far as we could discover, had anyone else. The idea of " participation magic " can therefore, as we see, spring spontaneously from the child's mind. T. showed just as much desire for the hearts of the various birds served at table as he did for the neck. In this case, however, he had a strong rival in J., so that there was always danger of a dispute if only one bird and therefore only one heart was on the table. T. gave as his reason for wishing to eat the heart that he would like to have two hearts. It was not so explicitly expressed as in the case of the neck, that he would like to acquire the forces resident in the heart. But it seems to us certain that a desire of this kind, even if not formulated in words, was a potent factor, for the heart was much more ardently desired than its tastiness alone would explain. This is also proved by the fact that a " substitute heart " which we offered in the form of some other piece of meat made heart-shaped was accepted and eaten with the same expression of special enjoyment. Only in T's case was this desire to eat the heart at all original. J. was obviously acting in imitation, without having the same motives as T. In order to avoid any dispute between the children about the heart we have more than once committed a pious fraud and manufactured a second heart. Moreover, one of us remembers quite distinctly, that when a child at home, both the heart and the tongue of the goose were greatly desired, simply because it was thought that special sources of power could be incorporated along with them.[1]

We give from our scientific diary one further example of magic thinking, this time concerning J. Father is sitting beside J., who is stroking his father's hand in a gentle loving way. Whilst doing so he accidentally scratches the back of his father's hand a little. J. is quite concerned at this and asks his father if it hurts, and then declares

[1] Is it not probable that the popularity of brains as a dish amongst some people may have a magical motive in the background ?

T

that the air—not he himself—has scratched his father. J. : " Is the air wicked ? " F. : " No, the air is not wicked." J. : " But why did it scratch with its finger ? " The finger scratched ; he himself did not intend it to, and so J. concludes that someone else must be guilty and falls back on personifying the wind. As Werner quite rightly points out, anthropomorphism is not the original element in such a case, but the original element is magical thinking, and it is only this which renders the anthropomorphism possible.

Werner interprets as magical the strict performance of certain series of actions by children who have become accustomed to them. He mentions this in connection with certain ceremonies which children perform on going to bed. We have not observed such ceremonies in our children, either when they went to bed or on any other occasion. As far as the retaining of definite sequences in performing actions is concerned, we can indeed trace the beginnings of such tendencies occasionally, but only after fixed habits had been laboriously instilled into the children. It is this very small degree of spontaneousness amongst the children in these cases, which speaks against Werner's interpretation. The observations have also no general applicability, for J., who in other respects tends much more strongly to magical thinking, showed himself far more independent of such tendencies to order than his elder brother. Finally the frequently observed tendency of trained and untrained animals to automatic behaviour also speaks against Werner's view, unless one is also willing to admit magical thinking in animals.[1]

Werner points out the difference between the magic of primitive peoples and that of children. The magic of primitive man is, he says, a fully developed form of life, the magic

[1] Fowls, which have been trained to get their food by roundabout means, go this roundabout way, even if their most direct way is made clear for them. The account of K. M. Schneider, " Einige Beobachtungen über die Ortsbeständigkeit bei Tieren," *Bericht über den 8. Kongress f. exp. Psychologie*, Jena, 1924, contains some informative details about the fixity of animal behaviour.

of the child only an insular formation within a cultural sphere of quite different shape. As opposed to this it may be pointed out that the children of primitive races have of course also a magical thinking which is quite different from that of the adult world.

Our observations have not yielded any evidence in support of Werner's claim that the child's magic is secret.

The child's magical thinking has been made comprehensible from the inevitable dependence of childish thinking on emotions. But the strongly emotionally determined thinking of the child is shown not only in cases where a decidedly magical method of thinking appears, when the reason is taken by surprise, but also in numerous other manifestations. The conversations which we have recorded give of course only a feeble representation of the real degree of emotions and feelings in the child's existence, because they almost all took place when the children were in a thoroughly balanced, level mood. Observation shows that the child's emotions are relatively much stronger than the adult's, but that they vanish much more quickly or change into another opposite emotion. So much attention has already been devoted by psychologists to the question of feelings and emotions in children, that there is no need to undertake a detailed examination here. We shall only include from the conversations a few details which were revealed about the content of the feelings and emotions of our children.

Firstly, we must once again point out that both children have a decided sense of humour. A grotesque figure like Pipo made an ineradicable impression on them (11). It was a real pleasure to hear the children laugh at humorous situations, freely and quite without restraint. Both children had a special sense for comic situations. The parents sometimes pretended to fight each other, and then the children's delight knew no bounds, and the combatants were urged on to new efforts. J. consoles himself for his father's absence with the thought that he will receive humorous accounts from him. We feel justified in saying that both children are superior to many children in their appreciation of wit and jokes and humour and we have done all we could to increase this gift which makes life so much easier.

There is very little to report concerning aesthetic experience in the children. They were very interested in looking at pictures, but it was solely the content which concerned them. It had to be something which gripped their imagination and afforded them the opportunity of occupying themselves further with it. What was the probable course of the story of which one episode was shown ? Coloured pictures were more popular than black and white ones. Wherever in the conversations the judgment " fine " (schön) is passed, it has the sense of " pleasant " or " desirable " or sometimes " interesting " or " attractive ". When T. finds the eyes of the Chinese " beautiful " (57) he probably means amusing or interesting.

The children were almost too fond of hearing their father sing songs, and they liked to hear instrumental music too. It is quite certain that music attracts the children more than the plastic arts. J. spontaneously expresses the desire to hear soldiers' songs again, which probably appealed to him especially because of his temperament, whilst T. declared that war songs make him sad (138). It has been frequently observed that children try to avoid unpleasant and sad situations and it can probably be said not merely of our own children, but quite generally, that the child's philosophy of life is to be termed optimistic, in so far as any such philosophic terminology can be accounted permissible in this connection.

(g) The Child as Psychologist.

From his earliest years the child is affected in his own way by the mood of the people of his surroundings, he reacts correspondingly to their expressive movements, but that of course does not imply that he is already in a position to make the psychological side of these events the subject of consideration. On the contrary the psychological apperception of the processes of the other person's consciousness is at first no concern of the child ; he manages without it, just as in the practice of everyday life the uneducated adult is much less familiar with psychological apperception than the psychologist would sometimes believe. When does the child begin to turn his attention towards psychological happenings as such ? Or let us ask the more specialized question, which is easier to answer : When does the child arrive at a psychological apperception of the processes of his own consciousness ? Our conversations furnish several notable contributions to this problem of self-observation (self-perception).[1]

We firstly mention again T's splendid remarks about colour-contrast (46) where we get the explanation of the phenomenon of the contrast in brightness as well as the observation itself. It seems as if the phenomena of colour-contrast and other optical phenomena most easily excite the child's psychological apperception. We may deduce this from the fact that most spontaneous utterances of children about the perception of experiences are concerned with the optical sphere. The sphere of sensory perception is also touched on in (51), but the psychological apperception is here stimulated by the mother, and the most that can be said is that the children follow the course of the argument with great attention. In the dreams we touch a central sphere of mental life, and T. is able to give reports about it in several conversations. Whenever a spontaneous account of a dream is given the dream must have become objective to the child, and this is especially clear in those cases in which a critical attitude is adopted towards the dream content. The cases where T. declares he must stop

---

[1] The problem of the development of self-observation in the child is dealt with in the following works. D. Katz, " Studien zur Kinderpsychologie," Leipzig, 1913 ; Carla Raspe, " Kindliche Selbstbeobachtung und Theoriebildung," *Zeitschr. angew. Psychol.*, vol. 23, 1924 ; G. Révész, " Ueber spontane und systematische Selbstbeobachtung bei Kindern," *Zeitschr. angew. Psychol.*, vol. 21, 1923.

to think whether he has done anything wrong or not, and where this thinking process can be successful, show that the child is already capable of the peculiar occupation with processes of internal events and their mastery, even if only at an elementary stage. The failure of such an attempt is quite definitely proved when T. in (123) declares that nothing occurs to him. In (134) we have a correct distinction made between two different internal attitudes which are related to one another, praying and speaking. It is worthy of note, that T. at times already shows a sense for what might be termed psychical causality. This is the case in (13), where a psychical law is noted. Here we may mention also what T. remarks (61) about a mnemotechnical process. T. seems to prove himself a supporter of the theory of non-sensual ideas in (58), where we are informed that thoughts cannot be seen. We will close these remarks, in so far as they deal with T., with a reference to the various occasions on which self-criticism is revealed. According to this T. is able not only to look back inwardly on his own thoughts and attitudes, but he is also able to raise himself above them in criticism.

As we have previously stated, J's utterances afford little or no material towards the problem of the child's perception of experience which we are discussing here. Indeed many of his remarks allow us to state with certainty that he regards psychical events as entirely bound to the physical. He regards the emotional movements of animals as equivalent to the expressive movements : " fishes aren't happy, they have no voice." We do not consider it a sign of psychological apperception when J.—this applies in a high degree to T.— shows an unreflective understanding of other people's behaviour, as for instance when he states that a small child must be treated with care (72). Referring to this understanding for other creatures, the behaviour of animals too is interpreted according to human standards. Indeed we find, as we had occasion to remark previously in another connection, the individual-psychological component of interpretation in J., when he, for instance, makes the monkeys play silly tricks.

With these last remarks we have touched upon the question of " understanding " from the point of view of the child in the sense in which this problem has been considered so frequently of late from the point of view of the adult. If, as is usual, understanding is compared with explaining, then we must say that the child is not capable of explaining a process along the lines of a superior general causal principle. It is probable that children of the age of our own have less a need for explanation than an endeavour to gain an understanding attitude. The understanding attitude is more primitive than the explanatory one. A glance at the behaviour of animals seems to prove this. The behaviour of the fellow-dog or the master will be somehow understandable to the dog, but who would speak here of behaviour which appears " explainable ? " The animal understands what takes place according to its expectation ; the unusual, which at first confuses it, is gradually overcome by habituation and becomes understandable in course of time. The same applies to a child at this age. The behaviour of the people of his surrounding is understood so far as it was expected, but if new conduct occurs then a relatively small amount of experience is needed to form a corresponding expectation, which is connected with that of the understanding.[1] Because of the preponderantly magical structure of childish thought the understanding behaviour of the child undergoes an extension far beyond the realm of animate objects (above all beyond his fellow creatures), to which it remains restricted in the case of the educated adult. Wherever the child interprets events in nature according to the principle of making, there is an understanding of these events of a quite different kind from that of the understanding of a person acting. The child's readiness to understand, his willingness to find sense interpretation is very much greater than the adult's. Even in children

[1] These observations are closely related to those of Heymans about intuitive psychology. *Zeitschr. Psychol.*, vol. 102, 1927.

of 10 years old this attitude is existent. What is to be expected from the understanding is shown by experiments of H. Reichner,[1] who showed to children two entirely different pictures in a stereoscope, binocularly merged into each other. The adult rejects the combination of a view of a city street and a hunting scene as completely absurd, but the child has no hesitation in discovering a reasonable sense in it. The child's tolerance in this experiment, and in others carried out according to different methods, is extremely large as compared with what the adult considers nonsensical. The child *wants* to understand, and as he feels no positive obstacles he does understand.[2]

(h) Social Psychology

The human beings who surround a child are much more important in an objective sense for his fate than the inanimate objects of his surroundings, and in the same way the child is doubtless occupied subjectively by them to a much greater extent than by the other factors in his world, including animals. Regarding it purely from the point of view of time, the child is, apart from short periods, in the company of human beings the whole day. He lives with them in the most familiar social intimacy and receives influences from them in a continuous stream, in return exerting his influence on them. We need not investigate here how the consciousness of another personality develops ; at all events at our children's present age it is already completely formed.

[1] Reichner, H., " Experimentelle und kritische Beiträge zur Psychologie des Verstchens," *Zeitschr. f. Psychologie*, vol. 104, 1927.

[2] J. Lindworsky in a small but suggestive work on causal thinking in primitive man, attempts to prove that the main root of the magical conception of the world is to be found in the tendency of primitive man to consider as clear and distinct many situations which the educated man recognizes not to be so. According to our remarks above, the child shares this tendency with primitive man. But in the child's case it is certainly not the only source from which his magical way of thinking flows. J. Lindworsky, " Die Primitiven und das kausale Denken," *Internationale Woche für Religions-Ethnologie*, Paris, 1926.

The social milieu in which our children moved was the household to which there belonged as constant members: the parents and grandmother, as relative constants, and the servants. In addition there were the chance visitors from amongst our circle of friends and acquaintances, both adults and children. Outside the house the children met other people at the kindergarten, when invited out, on walks, and when travelling. These were mainly children, and the meetings afforded the opportunity for merely fleeting social contacts. The social circle of children is not large, and the persons who come into the child's field of vision outside this circle are scarcely regarded as personalities, and are for the child an amorphous mass to a much greater extent than they are for adults, who actively seek social intercourse to a greater degree than do children.

Father and mother take pride of place in the social field of both children. This is a position of confidence which is quite unique. The children fly to them at night if disturbed by dreams; they must be told of everything the children have experienced, be it cheerful or sad; when they have told it, its reality is intensified. More than once a spontaneous declaration of love to their parents crosses their lips, and for this, very strange formulations may be chosen. When T. in conversation (92) declares that he cannot say how much he loves F. and M. we have already something of the experience that language fails in its task of expressing the strongest feelings. J. repeats the same thing as an imitation of what T. had shaped from his own experience. Whom do they love more, the father or the mother? Once T. states that he loves F. more, because he himself will become a Papa later, but that is really only an evasion, in order not to hurt M. In reality it is probable that the love towards both parents fluctuates; at times the parent present is loved more simply *because* he is present, at times the parent who is absent, because the child is yearning for him. But however strong the children's feelings towards the parents may be, it can happen that the parents

are completely forgotten, as for instance when the parents
have gone on a journey, or when the child is engaged in an
interesting pursuit. If the child is in the company of other
children and the parents come to take him home it may
be that the child pays no attention to the parents, who
are just treated like strangers. There should also not be
too many demands made for obvious proofs of the children's
love towards their parents. When the mother states that
she is very tired and would like to go to sleep, J. will not
permit it (135). He also demands that the mother should
be with her children more, and takes up a position against
his father on this point (136). It should scarcely be necessary
to protect this behaviour against psychoanalytical misinter-
pretations. It is not sexual jealousy which we see here
but the child's egoism, which is directed in the same
way against every other person, even if it is not his father.
Likewise, on another occasion it can be the father for whose
possession J. struggles against the mother. This kind of
egoism has receded somewhat in T. in consequence of his
greater age. When J. is a captain he intends to take on
board with him all the family because they were kind to
him as a child (94).

According to the variety of experiences undergone with
father and mother, the social attitudes of the children
towards the two are quite different. The father is the one
who is much better informed than the mother about handwork and technical things, and his person is endowed
with considerable importance by the fact that the positive
authority of the Psychological Institute with all its apparatus
is behind him, and the children are allowed to accompany
him to the Institute sometimes. And so he is the one to
turn to in all technical matters. Often the children are proud
of their father's profession, but occasionally they would
like him to be something else, as for instance a baker (119).
The father is the one who sometimes brings little things
back with him from his walks, and so he must be approached
in the attitude proper to the acquisition of toys and such-like

things. The father sings with the children, and therefore desires in this direction must be referred to him. And the mother ? She is known to the children as the place where bodily needs are attended to, she is the one who looks after food and clothing, she supervises hygiene and the division of the day. It is the mother principally who in the early years conveys the most important cultural values to the children, for she is with them much more than the father. She it is also who in the evening, at the most intimate part of the day, usually spends some time by their bedside and in mutual conversation looks back over the day's events. What the children learn about the earlier life of their parents also serves to make them take up differing attitudes towards them. In fact everything combines together to form round the father a social atmosphere value different from that of the mother.

Quite different social habitual attitudes are formed in the child in accordance with the varying social experiences which he undergoes with the various people of his surroundings. Other influences are the variety of the reactions with which he may or must react to his surroundings and finally the variety of the reactions to his own behaviour which he notices in his surroundings. Looking at the matter quite openly, we cannot speak of a general social attitude in a child in order to characterize him according to his social tendencies, but we must speak of a whole series of varying relations of the child towards the various people with whom he regularly comes into contact. These are chiefly the people in the family. The relationship towards father and mother has just been characterized. What is the children's attitude towards the grandmother ? Quite different from that towards the parents. The grandmother looks after the children when the parents are away on a journey or absent for a day or part of a day. Thus the children have in her presence a feeling of security which, however, is not so strong as that formed with respect to the mother. The grandmother also knows many stories which are intensely interesting to the children.   But the grandmother has never been able to acquire any great authority over the children ; it may be that the decreased physical elasticity of old age was responsible, for the children make no allowances for this.   It could be clearly observed that as the children grew older the grandmother's authority diminished ; probably girls, less lively than boys, would have been different in this respect. The conflicts with the grandmother, some account of which is furnished by the conversations, arose as a rule from the fact that the children thought the grandmother not sufficiently well-disposed to their play-desires and to the inevitable disorder in the nursery resulting from these desires.   In this connection the elder boy was more easily roused than the younger, whose whole relations to his grandmother must be accounted the happier. This relationship towards the grandmother is clear evidence that the values determining the social field are not constants but subject to continuous variation.

What is the relationship of the two children one towards the other ? They are attached to each other in an unusually intimate way.   They are very rarely separated from each other, they start the day together, play together, go for walks, and take their meals together, and they end the day together. If they are temporarily in different places, longing for each other soon sets in, in the younger boy's case stronger and more actively, in T's case less obviously but nevertheless unmistakably.   Only when they have certain common needs in social life can conflicts arise, in spite of their common interests, if the means at their disposal are limited.   This statement is also applicable to the relations of the two children one towards the other.   They play together, but the right of ownership of the presents they have received is still retained nevertheless. They borrow things from each other, but in the heat of the game they refuse to return them occasionally, and then we are perilously near to a conflict.

The rights of ownership are, however, strictly respected as a rule. They are extremely careful to see that each gets his own eating utensils at table, and that each gets his own cup offered to him, although the two drinking vessels are externally so similar that they are easily confused by other people. Being the elder, T. knows more, can do more, and performs more. Both boys feel this in their own way and J. strives to equal his brother. T. smiles sometimes when J. expresses naïve views, but it is not malicious, but rather good-humoured and is usually not felt to be offensive by J. By absolutely equal treatment of both children, and by special care, we have tried as far as possible to protect J. as the younger, from any feelings of inferiority. We think we have achieved our object, to the extent to which it can be achieved, but not entirely, as we recognize from J's greater efforts for recognition, which arise from his experiencing a by no means intended infringement on his personality by T. At various junctures in the conversations we were able to point out impulses of *manly protest* in J. This is obviously the psychological fate of the second child whose difference in age from that of the firstborn is not great enough to preclude emulative comparisons, as it is in the case of the father ; whose greater age is not felt as a disturbing element.

As no other relations lived in Rostock, the children only met them on occasional visits. But nevertheless they were treated with more intimacy than strangers, for the children had already heard so much about them from the parents, and received gifts and letters from them on birthdays and other similar occasions. The children themselves undertake a platonic increase of the family by frequently speaking about a baby which they would like. This baby must be a boy, so that it shall not cry and so that the children can play with it without having to be too careful. Even though the idea of relationship is sometimes judged by externals—father is allowed to kiss Uncle Julius his brother, because they are related (105)—yet the children do make a clearly recognizable difference in the treatment of those people who belong to the family and those who do not, under the influence of such experiences as the one in (76) where the grandmother does not run away as Elli did. Finally a not unimportant widening of the social milieu is performed by the workmen, shopkeepers, officials, etc., whom the children meet on various occasions. These acquaintances have clearly observable after effects in the numerous character-plays.

We have still to consider the social relationship of the children towards the servants and towards the playmates of about their own age. As we were endeavouring to bring out in our children the good points of the Montessori system, which seem to us to lie chiefly in the direction of educating to independence, we insisted that the children should be waited on as little as possible by the servants. The children themselves had to fetch and carry water, clear up what they spilled, tidy the play room, and perform any other similar jobs within their powers. By this we hoped—following Montessori—that the children would be taught not to look down on the household staff as ministering spirits, but would treat them in a friendly way. But how difficult it is to make the servants fall in with this plan, which is intended to be for their own social improvement. Thus we discovered repeatedly that they were beginning to wait on the children. It is therefore not surprising that the latter occasionally refused to perform some task, considering it the servant's affair. The social relationship of children to servants is essentially determined by the latter's capacity to understand the children in their games and elsewhere. What great differences exist in this respect was pointed out previously in the cases of Elli and Olga, but over and above this, the children here get to know for the first time a relationship of social superiority which is not determined by one's own capabilities or performances, but by the structure of the society in which the children are taking their places. Meetings with playmates of about the same age give the children the opportunity to preserve their own personalities. The children seem to have a very acute feeling for this.

Within the circle of children of about the same age we find the impulses to get oneself recognized by trying to gain either leadership or at least equality. Our children preferred friendships with boys; girls were only recognized if they were as rough as boys,[1] otherwise they were rejected. Appelschnut too is ridiculed more than once as a lady. It is only when he comes into contact with boys older than himself that T. develops ambition; he does not want his performances to lag behind those of his friends, other children must not be able to do anything better than he (60). It is well known that children are not fastidious in the choice of their friends, and this characteristic was also shown in our boys. However, occasionally a more deeply rooted friendship is observed, which seems to be based on the amount of agreement between the various qualities present. We did not observe any decidedly despotic relationships in our children's meetings with other children, neither in the sense that they themselves wanted to be despots nor that the other children played that part. A friendship was immediately struck up with two considerably older boys (97) because these boys know so well how to play with the children.

The numerous character-plays—and the conversations mention only a fraction of them—allow the child to imitate and shape as he pleases the social experiences which life has brought him, or the accounts of social conditions which he has learned from fairy-tales and other stories. In action and speech, in monologue and dialogue form, the most varied social situations are represented in the nursery. Thus here too we have a foretaste of later life with its multiplicity of social relationships, represented in a kind of serious play, without the children having however the slightest appreciation of the various social gradings of the different trades and professions.

[1] Groos reports as the result of an American questionnaire, that boys desired almost exclusively boys as playmates, and that girls were just as exclusive in their request for girls. K. Groos, *Die Spiele des Menschen*, Jena, 1899, p. 459.

3. CONSIDERATION OF THE FORM OF THE CONVERSATIONS

(a) The Conversational performance in its dependence on the mood of the child

What is true of us adults, that we are not always to the same extent in the mood for speaking and conversation, is also confirmed by the observation of children. The majority of the conversations recorded took place in the evening as the children were going to bed. This is in fact connected with circumstances which have nothing to do with the question of the importance of mood for the child's conversation, but the fact remains nevertheless, that the children show the greatest inclination for a more lengthy conversation in the evening. Seemingly it is not only their ethical receptivity which profits from the peculiar evening mood, but the intelligence too is more alert at this time of the day, the language shows a greater richness of expression, is at once more flowing and more concise. As in all other performances, the children are under the influence of a daily rhythm in regard to their capacity for linguistic expression and skill in speaking. We cannot of course trace this rhythm in every detail, but at least in many points. We have to some extent the opposite of the evening mood in the morning, immediately after waking up. The speaking and language machinery must so to speak get warmed up before it will function at full pressure. Both the children speak in the mornings noticeably more slowly and both speak less. As regards their mood immediately after waking a striking individual difference between the two children is to be noted. When J. opened his eyes and saw his parents a smile spread over his whole face, whilst T. usually displayed a somewhat sullen expression at first. If the two children had to waken at an unusual time J. thought nothing of it, but T. might take it very much amiss. There was a thoroughly catastrophic mood at the time when T. was accustomed to have his afternoon nap after lunch. When he awoke from this in such a mood, he might break out into seemingly meaningless fits of weeping. In the same way as the mood after waking, during the day the approach of tiredness was heralded by a disinclination to converse. The daily course of willingness to converse corresponds in its rise and fall approximately to the rise and fall of the physical state. This applies not only to the quantitative side of the conversations, but also to the quality of the performances. Feelings of great joy, which may be aroused by many unusual situations (journey by rail or ship, start of a walk which had been looked forward to) give wings to the child's conversation and cause speech performances which would be unthinkable at any other time (conv. 54). On the other hand physical indisposition such as precedes illness, or even the illness itself, especially if it is a feverish one, can reduce the child's performances in all respects and also as regards conversation, indeed it can even temporarily put the child back years. In view of such experience, which not only we, but all child psychologists have had on occasion, it should be made a rule that whenever there is any striking decline in a child's performances a medical examination should be resorted to. Often inflamed tonsils or some other disturbing change in the physical state will give an explanation of a psychologically inexplicable change in a child's behaviour.

We have proved that during illness to some extent an earlier and seemingly long passed level of mental development reappears and makes its presence felt again. The fact that the mental structure is composed of layer after layer is made particularly clear during illness, but it may also be noted, naturally in a less pronounced form, during normal health. Also on days when he is in perfect health the child's performances as a whole fluctuate round an average commensurate with his age. For under favourable influences the child produces performances which will be possible only very much later as average performances, and when conditions are not favourable he descends to maximum performances which were his average some considerable time previously. The performances in conversation under discussion here are also affected by this general law. It is only in theory that we can get clear-cut divisions between stages of mental development from various graduated ages; personal experience shows how these stages work through and against one another, governed in their development by the above mentioned apsychonomic factors as well as by others.[1]

(b) Extent of the sentences in the child's conversation and remarks on style

As early as the test-series of Binet and Simon, which were adopted later by other authors, the testing of the child for his capacity to repeat accurately a sentence of definite length said to him has enjoyed a certain popularity. For instance the five-year-old child is asked to say a sentence of ten syllables, the six-year-old one of sixteen without error. It is well known of course that these performances give no indication of the length of the sentences which the children are able to produce spontaneously in conversation. Our dialogues can make some contribution to the question of the amount by which spontaneous sentences

[1] With reference to the world of perception, E. R. Jaensch in his numerous works on this subject has taken up the attitude that there is a layer-like structure and a counter-action of the layers, one against the other. Werner in a similar fundamental attitude points out that a human being possesses not only one mental attitude simply or one layer of experience and reaction, but that one and the same person appears at different times to belong to genetically different stages. (Werner, p. 30.) Elsa Köhler was struck by the fact that Annchen when excited made many speech mistakes, a fact which fits without difficulty into the method of consideration adopted here, in so far as excitement lowers the level of performance capacity. (E. Köhler, p. 203.)

are longer than these test-sentences. What is the extent of sentences which are produced by the children in the dialogues ? The limit of the lowest level is reached with the one-word sentences made up of the particles " yes " and " no ", but the highest limit is not so easy to determine. In many of the children's utterances it is very difficult to decide what is to be regarded as a sentence unit, for at times sentence units are strung one after the other without any speech pause, yet each could be properly regarded as an independent unit, whereas on the other hand parts of sentences are uttered, separated by speech pauses, and the child probably considers these parts as speech units. In this respect, the method of dividing the parts of the children's speech adopted by us in the dialogues and revealed externally by the various punctuation marks, is not entirely free from a certain arbitrariness. But we feel on the whole that we have made the divisions correctly. Proceeding from this division we might undertake a statistical investigation into the frequency of two- three- and four-word sentences, etc., but we fear that the result obtained would not be in any way proportionate to the labour expended. In general it may be said that the length of the sentences formed by T. in his speeches does not vary to any great extent from that of sentences which the adult would form under the same circumstances. This may be seen from the fact that our own utterances in the dialogues do not materially differ in length from those of T. It also seems to be certain that the sentences formed by J. are inferior in length to those of his elder brother. Over and above these general details we can state one definite statistical fact. In the conversations T. utters quite indubitably sentence units of thirty to forty words, and these are not rare exceptions. The longest sentences produced by J. also, but more rarely, attain this notable extent. In view of such findings, which can scarcely be isolated examples, it is impossible to agree with Kroh in the following statement : " The six-year-old prefers sentences of three to five words, although longer sentences also occur." [1] How halting and jerky a conversation with T. would have been if he had preferred sentences of three to five words.

It was not within the scope of this work to undertake statistical investigations about the use of various types of sentences and about the vocabulary used by the children, because these problems belong rather to the technique of children's language and have been frequently investigated.[2] The stock of words used by T. exceeds the average found in children of his age and is probably connected with his passionate love of books (fairy-tales, *Robinson Crusoe*, Scharrelmann's *Berni*, etc.) which he has read aloud to him and from which he adopts good linguistic expressions. He has more than once surprised us by his use of them in appropriate places. T. has a keen sense for beautiful language and a good memory for impressing it on himself. J's vocabulary probably does not exceed that of a child of his age and social level.[3]

There are hardly any Mecklenburg dialect words to be found in the children's conversations. The local dialect has had a much greater influence phonetically on the children's speech. Apart from the word " pestol " in conv. (1) we have not discovered any radical new creations.[4] The " perlicke perlacke " of conv. 124 is also worthy of further mention. Here we have the beginnings of onomatopœic linguistic creation, even though the starting point is this pretended magic-word.

[1] O. Kroh, " Zur Psychologie des Grundschulkindes," *Württembergische Schulwarte*, i, 26.

[2] Cf. W. Boyd, " The development of sentence structure in Childhood," *British Journal of Psychology*, vol. 17, 1927.

[3] Cf. in this connection Joh. Schlag, " Häufigkeitsproben aus dem Sprachschatz von 6–8 jährigen Kindern," *Pädagogisch-psychologische Arbeiten*, Leipzig, 1921, vol. 9.

[4] An investigation is at present being carried out into the question of the extent to which children can be incited to the invention of *radical* new expressions for objects whose names they do not know. Linguistic analogical formations are of less interest.

(c) *General mental attitudes, and the children's questions in the conversations*

In connection with some peculiar ideas propounded by Betz, Bühler adopted the method of referring to general intellectual ways of behaviour in rather strange language as the " thoughy " " butty " " neverthelessy " behaviour of a person.[1] An analysis of the mental attitudes of the child in conversation to a certain extent conforms and even extends what Bühler has done. In conversation with adults the child inwardly takes up very varied attitudes, the most important of which we will mention, though without any hope of doing justice to all their different nuances.

The distinguishing of active and reactive attitudes makes possible the first rough orientation. By reactive attitudes we mean the child's forms of reaction to the influence of the conversation-partner, and by active attitudes those which are revealed in the child's attempts to influence the conversation-partner. It must be noted, however, that both attitudes remain in the last resort conditioned by the presence of an adult conversation-partner.

Active attitudes are shown by the child firstly in all questions which he addresses to the adult in order to stimulate him to a reply, and then in all the child's assertions, proposals, wishes, requests, and demands. Let us begin with the child's questions, and endeavour to get some sort of order into their multifarious varieties of meaning. When the question has been asked, the child is awaiting information which in most cases will satisfy his mental need. The question is the real expression of seeking in the mental sphere, corresponding to the groping movements of the physical organs in the external world. The child asks the questions boldly because he is still in the happy position of believing that there is no question which cannot be answered by the adult. The discovery of this belief

[1] Bühler, p. 392.

brings out in another form what we have previously
mentioned, namely that a child would scarcely ask a question
about a subject, however remote, unless this subject were
present to him in some form or other—frame it as indefinitely
as one will—that is to say in some schematic anticipation.[1]
If a question is asked about the entirely unknown name of
an object noticed for the first time, then the existence of
a name must surely be presumed, and if the reason for a
process noticed for the first time is asked, then the validity
of some general law governing the process, even though
it be a magical one, is surely presumed and so on. Looked
at from the standpoint of the adult, the scheme the child
tries may be quite false, but that is not important : what
really matters is the fundamental fact that any scheme at
all is present, which demands completion.   Only circumstances which lie quite outside the child's interest, and therefore in a certain sense outside his world, do not appear
" questionable " to him, and so cannot be included in any
scheme, however vague.   The commonest question which
occurred is seen in (32) " How shall I ask then ? "   Thus
a scheme for questioning is sought.

The use of the most important interrogative particles
makes it seem probable that the child is capable of understanding the most usual categories of questioning. We can
group the child's questions into two main classes : those
caused by the behaviour of the conversation-partner,
where the question is caused either by a verbal utterance
of the adult or by some behaviour, which the child would
like explained, and those which are asked apparently quite
spontaneously, without any external stimulus being recognizable. We should then logically speak of spontaneous questions. It was rare that a question from the adult immediately

[1] Here we may be allowed to quote the last statement of reproductive
thinking given by Selz, " In reproductive thinking the question acts . . .
as, an incomplete knowledge-complex, like a blank cheque, in which at
least one of the parts to be filled in is lacking. In the question formulated
the missing part is characterized categorically by the interrogative
particles : What, where, when, how much ? etc. *Kantstudien*, vol. 32, 1927.

elicited one from the child in return, as for instance in (66) where in response to F's question " Do you know where Eskimos carry their children ? " T. asks " Where ? " They are quite in the minority as compared to the cases when the child makes his question dependent on a statement by the adult. An entirely independent and clear category is formed by those questions in which the explanation of a word is demanded : What does elect mean ? (140). What does permission mean ? (140). We can also distinguish as a separate category those questions to which the child himself knows the answer, and by which he wishes to discover if the adult does also. Examples : T. asks his new friends if they know his father's name (97). We may also mention the conundrum-questions. What is bigger than an elephant but it is not an animal and not a human being ? (38). The child does not ask the conundrum-question because of intellectual confusion, but on the contrary he is trying for his own amusement to bring the adult into confusion, and reveals a roguish delight if he apparently succeeds. There is also a clearly-defined category of questions in which inquiry is made about the existence of persons, animals, or things, although of course it is obvious that the child's thinking attaches a different meaning to the word " existence ". Examples : Are there really any dwarfs ? (21). Are there any real negroes ? (21). Did Robinson Crusoe really live ? (134). A separate group is formed by the questions about past and future events, concerning both themselves and others. They are much more numerous than the other special categories of questions mentioned. Examples : Did Papa fight Goliath ? (20). What are you giving Papa for his birthday ? (129). May I sleep in your bed ? (123). Will you buy me some goldfish ? (127). As shown by the last examples quoted, the expression of the child's wishes here takes place in the form of questions. Much more numerous again than the category of questioning just mentioned are those with a causal and final tinge. Examples : Why did you stay in Berlin and not go back to that school ?

(19). Why are negroes really black then ? (63).—Just as the cause and purpose of an event may be asked about so can also its course, its " How " be made the subject of inquiry. Admittedly a strict division of the child's questions from the causal and final ones is not always easy here. We quote only quite definite examples : How does the calf drink from the cow ? (38). How does one cook with this book ? (16). How does the earth turn ? (79). How are elephants caught ? (24). Questions about the time and place of events and actions are also very numerous. Examples : Where do shop-assistants live ? (68). Where was the giant born ? (122). When did Goliath live ? (23). When did Papa's parents die ? (116). Questions about the origin and beginnings of things take up much space in the conversations. The contents of everything that we proved previously to belong to the world of the child can become the subject of the child's questions about its origin and the way in which it came into being. It is especially easy in these questions about the origin of things for the child to proceed from question to question, each one leading farther away from the original theme, so that we may here speak quite accurately of chains of questions. Unsatisfied by the information he has just received, but at the same time affected by it, the child in his urge for investigation goes farther and father back into the history of a thing's beginnings ; at last the person he is questioning has to recognize that no end to these regressive questions is to be hoped for, and he closes the inquisition by some suggestive turn which seems proper to him. In our experience it is not rare to meet with chains of questions of ten links, which were brought to a close by the adult, without the child having shown any inclination to stop of his own accord. Many of these chains of questions give the impression that it is not merely the child's urge for knowledge which is the determining factor, but that there is also a joy in the form and the progression of the rhythm question-answer, question-answer, which partakes of the character of a game.[1] It seems reasonable to suggest this, especially when the later questions of a chain, which started well, noticeably sink to a lower intellectual level. But we have a considerably more disciplined performance than in the commonplace succession of a chain of questions when as in several conversations an accumulation of questions touches on the same subject after approaching it from different angles, or when the questions are devoted to various subjects, one after the other. A count has shown that in our 141 conversations about 300 questions are asked by both children. These questions are, however, not uniformly distributed over the individual conversations, but quite the reverse. There are many conversations in which the children ask no questions at all, and there are others in which questions accumulate, without, however, becoming a chain of questions in the sense defined above. Thus, for instance, conversations 19, 20, and 140 contain respectively 9, 16, and 26 questions (19 by T. and 7 by J.). It may be assumed from this that there is a tendency to perseveration, once the child has got into a questioning attitude. This is revealed in numerous questions, one following on the other, where the questions already asked have the effect of strengthening the perseverative attitude. Among the child's mental attitudes in conversation already observed there is scarcely any other which tends so strongly towards perseveration as this questioning attitude. It is quite certain that this is connected with the child's unlimited need of expansion. In the child's questions there are revealed confusions and uncertainties of varying

[1] From the available literature we quote the following example of regressive questions. Conversation between Clara and Günther Stern : What does that one eat ? Fishes.—Why does it eat fishes ? Because it is hungry.—Why doesn't it eat bread ? Because we don't give it any.— Why don't we give it any ? Because the bakers only bake bread for human beings.—Why not for fishes ? Because there isn't enough flour.— Why isn't there enough flour ? Because enough corn doesn't grow. You know flour is made of corn.—Oh yes ! (Stern, p. 143.) Regression is also an art-form of the fairy-tale and folk-song. Might it not have received stimulus from children's conversation ?

degrees. When T. asks in conversation (100) the alternative question, whether the child is a boy or a girl, he is naturally counting on the fact that either the one thing or the other must be the case. And the situation is similar in all the cases in which the child may expect the question he asks to be answered either in the affirmative or in the negative. Questions referring to well-known and familiar objects, persons, or events have quite a different structure from those which refer to unknown and unfamiliar ones, and which, therefore, are intended to conquer new territory. It may be said that the latter questions have a greater degree of freedom. The blank-cheques (to use the very appropriate analogy of Selz) which the child fills in with his questions, have, therefore, a very different standard of filling in. This could easily be demonstrated in detail from the questions in the material we ourselves have accumulated, but this specialized investigation would go far beyond the scope of our investigation into the problem of question. We must limit ourselves to what has already been said about the questions of the child, and turn to other mental attitudes of the child which are revealed in the conversations.

In the immediate vicinity of the real questions, which are easily recognizable from their external form, we meet the interrogative assertions of the child. These are utterances which appear as categorical opinions, but where the child's tone of voice usually betrays that they are being placed before the adult in order to induce him to pass judgment on the child's own opinions, whether it be one of approval or condemnation. We give one example of many. After the conversation about dwarfs in (21) T. says to M. " Oh, but I'll grow ". We see clearly that the statement has here the character of an interrogative assertion (and at the same time of a wish) from the fact that T. asks another question as soon as he has had confirmation from his mother that he will grow : " How can you tell ? " There are all kinds of transitions from the interrogative assertion to the categorical statement, which the child demands to have recognized by the adult. Both in external form and in internal structure these categorical opinions of the child are the rule in our conversations. All others, including even that of interrogative assertion represent the exceptions. We counted above amongst the active attitudes of the child those which are expressed in proposals, wishes, requests, and commands. J. makes a demand in conversation 18 when he turns to his father with the words " Sing the song of the burnt boy ". In conversation 91 J. expresses numerous wishes about his approaching birthday, and T. makes a request in conversation 7 : " Mama, I want to have a guide-book."

We will describe a few reactive attitudes of the child in conversation amongst which, according to what we have said above, we understand those which were taken up under the influence of the conversation-partner. When the parents give information there is usually complete insight into the contents of the information. These cases form the great majority of the reactive attitudes. Example : If a doctor says so, then it is so, for a doctor knows everything (123). We come to the attitude of mental opposition, which can run through all stages from the gentlest, scarcely noticeable objection to the open contradiction, obstinately maintained. To M's encouraging remark " you must want to, then you will be able to " T. modestly objects " Not as quickly as all that " (conv. 13). There is little readiness to accept information in conversation 32. T. asks why people didn't come before animals. M. : " It just was so, one can't ask why." T. : " How shall I ask then ? " The opposition is a little more determined in T's words : But Papa did *almost* fight him (conv. 20). In conversation 21 we meet a still stronger insistence on a standpoint taken up. Here T's own opinion that negroes are quite different from white people is maintained in three succeeding sentences. (1) But I'm sure they've different habits from us. (2) They show their teeth when they laugh. (3) But they do have other habits. They say " hee hee " when they laugh. We get objection and disappointment together in T's words " You shouldn't say things like that, it's rude " (conv. 53). If we compare T's opposition attitudes with those of J., our impression is that those of the younger child are less concrete but more governed by the emotions and therefore more definitely subjective. As comparisons we give some examples for J. J. : " Does straw grow in meadows too ? " M. : " No, grass grows in meadows." J. : " No, I've seen straw growing in meadows " (conv. 30). What obstinacy J. develops in conversation 81, in order to get into T's bed ! But J's strongest opposition, admittedly produced experimentally, is to be found in conversation 27, concerning the identity of T.

All the mental attitudes in conversation which we have distinguished, and all others which might perhaps be distinguished, are determined by factors of social psychology. They arise in the social sphere from the interplay between adult and child. Even though this proves that the adult plays his part in the development of the conversation we should like to deal with this point separately and in more detail. The attitudes adopted by the adult in conversation are at one time active and at another reactive, just as the child's attitude was shown to be. But the adult does not need to be so active towards the child as the child does towards the adult, nor does the adult lose himself in reaction to the child to the same extent as the child usually loses himself to the adult. If a dialogue is proceeding between two adults who are of about the same intellectual level, then the swing to and fro between active and reactive attitudes is much more pronounced. If two adults are building up a conversation under these conditions, neither of the two will be able to prophesy with certainty the course of the conversation. It is like a game of chess, where, granted equal skill in the participants, the course of the game is determined by the reciprocal strategy and tactics of the players. The more superior one player is to the other the more does he " play " with his opponent. In a dialogue the intellectually superior conversation-partner has control over the development of the conversation. He gives his partner just as much freedom and causes him just as much confusion as he likes. In the same way the adult in conversation with the child has the course of affairs almost completely in his power. The only difficulties which the child can cause the adult are of pedagogical nature. How shall he answer in order to make himself intelligible to the child's small comprehensive capacity and store of experience, and yet at the same time be subjectively satisfactory to the child? Everyone is not capable of unbending and looking at things from the child's point of view. Of course, even in conversation with an adult one will adapt oneself to the individuality and personal situation of the partner concerned in order to be understood, but when conversing with an adult it will be very rare for pedagogic adaption to have to go as far as is necessary when dealing with a child.

The adult will respond to the child's questions as far as possible. His replies can either satisfy the child completely, and so end the conversation, or they can give the impulse to new questions. Even when very extensive tolerance is exercised towards the child's free conduct of the course of the conversation, the adult will yet be obliged to intervene occasionally, when the child is beginning to wander from the point. Then the adult must call him to order, i.e. to the subject. The adult must also at times give a fresh impetus to the conversation when he notices that the child's energy is flagging and is no longer able of itself to undertake a new flight up from the level of the conversation. The adult can also to a large extent control the time he will spend on an old theme and when he will pass on to a new one. It also depends on him in a large measure where and when he will round off the conversation.

(d) Concerning some aspects of the form of the child's
thinking

When we were considering magical thinking we pointed
out that this form of thinking, which was rooted pre-
eminently in the field of emotion, is accompanied by a calm
and objective form which is destined to take precedence
over it stage by stage and gradually to expel it completely.
The real task imposed on child psychology by general
psychology, is to describe how the child's thinking frees
itself from emotional fetters and approaches the ideal of
pure objectivity in a series of conquests of various obstacles
and mistakes. Without making any claim to completeness,
a claim which is fulfilled in the investigations of other authors
into this subject, we intend to point out here some of the
stages in the development of the child's thinking towards
the ideal goal, or really, more correctly, we shall point out
from our conversations some of the obstacles to this development. Magical thinking is not sufficiently characterized
by being described as emotional, but only becomes such
by the addition of special animistic forces in order to make
events understandable, forces to which the child's emotion
gives birth. But even the child's emotion, which does not
lead to magical thinking, often enough causes the act of
thinking to miss its goal. The proposition of the excluded
third applies only to the harmonious logic of the adult and
not to the child's emotional thinking. Otherwise T. could
not have replied in answer to the question which of various
things he liked best, that he liked everything best (1).
The fact is he is intensely pleased with everything. The
joyful emotion admits of no selection of superlatives. And
a second opposite example from the same conversation :
J. finds the same book at once naughty and nice because
although the book's behaviour has aroused his displeasure
he does not want to say anything which might offend it.
The book has an ambivalent character. Stern thinks that
the child has no need of verification as long as he thinks

egocentrically.   But thinking egocentrically means being
greatly subject to the emotions.   We found this statement
confirmed by Stern in numerous cases.

Groos (loc. cit,. p. 172) has pointed out that we meet with
a loosely-connected series of associations in many children's
processes of thought, similar to those met with in the
meaningless rapid series of ideas of maniacs.   In our discussion of the individual conversations we were able to
point out numerous cases of the type Groos has in mind ;
we referred to them as flat associative thinking.   We hope
that this expression, which was intended to prejudice as
little as possible, in theory has not been misunderstood,
and we should like to add the following details concerning
its use.   If it is believed that the laws of association are
not exclusively able to make ordered higher thinking
understandable, but that somewhat in Ach's sense determinative tendencies are to be included, or that according to
Selz the laws of ordered thinking are the expression of the
constant correlations within a system of specific reactions,
it must also be admitted that at least in a subsidary sphere
of the movement of ideas, events take place with more or
less extensive approach to external associations, and that these
act more effectively on the child and may even be revealed
in the adult in occasional relapses, as for instance in a rapid
series of ideas in meaningless order.   Mental development
means then a more and more extensive liberation from
the associative in favour of the admittedly superior principle
of ordered thinking.   Bühler means this emancipation when
he (p. 415) speaks of an increase in the heteronomy of
thinking with the child's increase in age.   By classing many
of the terms in the conversations as " decidedly associative "
we meant to make it clear to supporters of a non-associa-
tionist theory, that in the turns concerned a relapse into
the associative has taken place, a relapse which was no
longer the rule.   But if anyone is a supporter of a constellation theory in G. E. Müller's sense then he must understand our expression to mean that contrary to the

expectation that the constellation would become effective, it fails and associations proceeding from it break through the order and cause the real goal of the thinking to be missed. According to this explanation it will be understood what we mean by the statement that all J's utterances are more powerfully determined by association than those of T. External attachment plays a strikingly important part for instance in J's utterances in (9) and (41). We regard it also as the effect of a purely external attachment when in numerous conversations, questions and statements are strung together which are connected not materially, but by a common feeling. We still have to discuss the general importance of associative tendencies for the manner in which the child conducts his conversations.

The following logical false performances which could also be classed as associative slips may serve to illustrate further the more general remarks outlined above. T. asks if there is not a shooting-moon, and he is led to this idea by " shooting-star " which he already knows (34). Nevertheless there could be shooting-moons, and so the associatively produced performance is a parapraxis only from the standpoint of the adult with his greater experience. The following are, however, not so easily excused. T. asks whether a lost property office exists for the limbs people have lost by amputation (112). An observation of the fixed connection between the limbs and the body ought to have prevented T. from assuming that human limbs could be lost like things which are not so closely connected with the body and that they could be obtained once more from the lost property office. When T. turns a caterpillar into a wild animal because of a similarity in sound (113) we have an associative slip, from which T. should have been saved by a look at the harmless creature. But at the same time that T. can fall a victim to analogical thinking he has on the whole mastered it thoroughly, as we see from conversation 54 with its numerous and surprisingly appropriate analogies between the parts of a railway train and human features. Whereas the cases quoted exhaust almost all the parapraxes of this kind committed by T. They are so numerous in J. that it is impossible to quote them all individually. He furnishes a classic example in his fusion of " Ohrläppchen " and " Waschläppchen " (135).

T's confusion of lie and mistake (42) is to be explained not as purely associative, but as a misunderstanding of conceptual conditions, and the same applies to his statement that he doesn't want a strange wife (3). T's questions as to whether Berlin and the king were " discovered " (74, 80) reveal the uncertainty prevailing about these by no means easy concepts. The concreteness of the child's thinking has often been pointed out. The simplicity and uniformity of thinking in the perceptual makes up the sense and meaning of so-called concrete thinking (Werner, p. 141). J. takes it literally that the meat is covered with water, when his mother has only read it to him (1). J. makes no distinction between writing and drawing (9). T's thinking shows much less of this concreteness ; it is a good performance to declare that thoughts cannot be seen (58).

Other child psychologists have investigated the development of causal thinking. Our conversations also provide some material towards the question of how it is prepared. The frequently repeated idea of a connection between the colour of the skin and temperature may be mentioned in this connection (63, 66, 96). The idea : if people don't go for a walk they die (59) is lapidary. Here we may once more refer to the discovery of a function between the degree of love towards a person and the warmth of their hand (62). When T. draws conclusions from the agreement of two clocks as to the greater probability of correctness compared with another clock showing a different time (47) we have a true induction, which is not admitted by Stern's general principle that the child knows neither induction nor deduction, but only transduction. But our experience leads us to agree with Stern that the form he terms syncretism is frequently to be met with in the child's thinking.

*(e) Association, perseveration and other tendencies which
determine the course of the child's conversation*

The dialogue between an adult and a child is a structure in the creation of which, as has been repeatedly said, both conversation-partners are engaged in their own way. The explanation of the form of a dialogue would therefore include of necessity a thorough analysis of the adult's performance and a determination of its formulative power. At the beginning of this work we pointed out the extent to which any explanation of the child's utterances must suffer from the lack of certain preliminary work in general psychology, and this deficiency is revealed as an even greater obstacle to the explanation of the utterances of the adult. There is no generally recognized theory of thinking, much less a theory of dialogue which can satisfy a theory of thinking, however efficient it may be. Dialogue presents a problem in social psychology in which thinking only occupies one side, important as that side is.

Without a phenomenology of dialogue a theory of dialogue is quite without foundations, for, as everywhere, it is true here too that we must first discover what it is before we can say how it is to be explained. We could not consider it within the scope of this work to write a complete phenomenology of dialogues, for it would have gone beyond the limits we had set ourselves and the material would have had to be considerably increased by the addition of dialogues between adults. Nevertheless numerous observations scattered through the whole work contain the elements of a phenomenology of dialogue which we hope will prove reliable and helpful for future more penetrating investigations into this subject. The observations alluded to are chiefly those with regard to the child's mental attitudes in conversation, and those concerning dialogue as a unit resting or developing between the participants in the conversation.

Dialogue is a phenomenon of social psychology, and

thinking plays a predominant part in it. What is the situation as regards the possibility of utilizing the results obtained by the thought-psychologist in order to explain the form of our dialogues ? We would be the first to acknowledge the valuable results obtained in thought-psychology in the last few years, but for our particular purpose these results cannot be utilized because the thinking performances which have been investigated are, almost without exception, artificial productions lacking the natural conditions of growth and set in motion by the will of the person conducting the experiment. The assumption that thinking under these conditions took place in forms which were essentially the same as in actual life, even if slightly simplified ought to have been subjected to a rigorous investigation whereas it was taken for granted. In reality the conditions of laboratory experiment chosen restricted normal thinking considerably and precluded certain types of behaviour, first and foremost all genuinely unrestricted spontaneous thinking processes. Where, in experiments on thinking carried out up to the present, can we find for instance all these mental attitudes of conversation of which we have spoken above—and we are far from believing that we have grasped and included all those which actually occur ? These attitudes can only grow in the absolute freedom of a dialogue which takes place naturally. The physicist is justified in assuming immediately that laboratory conditions leave the course of events so unaffected that the laboratory experiment must give an indication of the natural course of events, but the psychologist may not make this assumption. The contrast between processes of thinking in laboratory experiments, as they have been carried out up to the present, and processes of thinking in normal life, which is our aim, may perhaps be made clearer to many people by means of a contrast of a similar kind in another sphere of psychology, namely that of perception. It was also a mistake to proceed as was previously done in the investigation of the sense of touch, by investigating the pressure and spatial thresholds and similar " simplified " sensations of touch, expecting by this means to arrive at the tactual performances of everyday life, as for instance the cloth dealer and the housewife who tests his goods know them.[1] The measures taken in the laboratory at these investigations into touch usually precluded those tactual sensations which have grown naturally, and which are of an entirely different structure from those previously produced in the laboratory. We are of the opinion that the thought-psychology of the laboratory has in the same way, up to the present, also precluded certain forms of thinking of everyday life, indeed probably just the most important forms. Usually the experiments were performed with nonsense syllables, on which the subject, after instruction, had to perform certain operations. Even where the experiments were performed with meaningful material or with whole meaningful sentences it could hardly be claimed that the subject revealed spontaneousness. The same must also be said of the valuable and ingenious investigations of Selz, whose results we were in part able to utilize. Not without reason Koffka remarks regarding these investigations " Selz has devoted a great deal of acumen and an immense amount of pains to the answering of such questions. But one important thing he has not taken into account : he is attempting to investigate thinking and indeed productive thinking, with the aid of tasks which are by nature fundamentally different from true, living, productive thinking ".[2] The above remarks are of course not directed against the experiment in thought psychology, but are intended only to emphasize the necessity of making good its deficiencies in certain directions.

Köhler's experiments on anthropoid apes have provided us with important contributions towards the psychology of spontaneous thinking, and we have previously referred to their fundamental importance. But the results were

[1] In reference to this cf. D. Katz, *Der Aufbau der Tastwelt*, Leipzig, 1925.
[2] K. Koffka, " Bemerkungen zur Denkpsychologie," *Psychologische Forschung*, vol. 9, p. 164 ff., 1927.

obtained from animals which have no speech and not from human beings in dialogue, whose organs of speech possess such a decisive importance for the course of thinking, since it is they which further social contacts. The special features of many of the problems here presented were seen by Wertheimer [1] and Koffka, but in both these scholars the empirical basis is narrow and there has been no attempt made by either to transfer them to the sphere of social psychology.

Since the state of affairs is as described above, it may be deemed quite hopeless to try to explain satisfactorily all the tendencies of form which determine the course of conversation. We will content ourselves with mentioning some of them, beginning with the best known, the associative and perseverative tendencies. Koffka has gone farthest in his opposition to the association theory of the course of ideation and the process of thinking. He will not admit the effect of association alone even in the case of mechanical learning. " If I have learned pum lap mechanically, even then the theory of mere external association is false. In this case also I have created a uniform complex, a pair, usually iambic or trochaic, that is, with a specific dynamic force in which admittedly there cannot be much sense, i.e. whose total congruent law requires only a loose material connection. Lap is not the opposite of pum and does not stand in any other logical relation to it, but nevertheless it belongs to it, let us say as its colleague. The fact that just these two syllables have become colleagues is quite arbitrary but it is not for nothing that the learning of such nonsense syllables is such an unpleasant business. . . . " [2] We may agree with this point of view and yet be of the opinion that external association is an indispensable factor in psychology, and that we can dispense with it as a liminal

---

[1] M. Wertheimer, (1) *Über das Denken der Naturvölker, Zahlen und Zahlgebilde* ; (2) *Über Schlussprozesse im produktiven Denken*. Erlangen, 1925.

[2] K. Koffka, " Psychologie. Lehrbuch der Philosophie," *Die Philosophie in ihren Einzelgebieten*. Edited by M. Dessoir, Berlin.

concept just as little as perceptual psychology could dispense
with the concept of sensation as a liminal concept. If there
are introduced together into the consciousness two thought-
contents, between which the inner connections are as small
as possible, then approaching as near as possible to the
liminal case, reproduction by means of mechanical association takes place. On numerous occasions in the individual
discussions we spoke about the associative appearance of
a new theme, and by this we meant an appearance governed
not by inner, meaningful, logical connections, but by an
association which was to a large extent senseless. What
we mean here is quite clear in all the conversations
governed by the situation and in many which are bound
to it, where the sequence of themes is determined by
what the child sees as his gaze moves casually across
his field of vision.   But the meaningful significant use
the child makes of these themes, suggested by association,
is quite another matter. Both what has already been
said about the associative determination of themes, and
that which still remains to be said, apply in general to
what rises perseveratively as a theme into the child's
consciousness. There is a difference only in so far as perseverative, i.e. spontaneous ideas as a rule cause an alteration
of the theme whereas association, by reproducing new sides
of the theme can often cause the child to linger over them.
We have pointed out above the useful purpose which perseveration is able to perform in conversation, and the same
applies to pure association. Both processes of reproduction,
although logically neutral, can yet become constructive
factors in the conversation ; if they are not ruled by the sense
and if they themselves rule, they change into destructive
factors by causing a departure either from the theme itself
or from its meaningful-logical treatment.

What happens then to a theme which has been prepared
for either associatively or perseveratively ? It may lead
the child to simply innumerable quite different treatments,
which, however, being meaningful are no longer subordinated

only to the purely associative-perseverative sphere. Innumerable are the forms by which the child frees himself from the restraint of the effect of events, external in the liminal case. When the child has a mastery of speech to the extent our children had, the fact that he can express in speech the same contents at different times and in different ways proves that the emancipation from pure association has begun. If someone crosses the street and catches sight of the works of Kant displayed in a shop window, the reproduction of the idea of Kant which takes place because of this sense perception is as accidental as anything well can be. But if the person concerned sets up meaningful intelligent considerations as a result of it, whether he immediately embarks on a recapitulation of Kant's philosophy, or tells the person accompanying him about the philosopher of Königsberg, in each case we have sensible performances, no longer to be understood as merely associative. What a child makes of a theme need not maintain the same high level as the fictitious performance of an adult reproduced above, but it nevertheless remains sensible. It is meaningful when the child makes a sensible statement about the theme based on his previous experiences, or when he formulates a skilful question in order to learn further details, or when he allows his imagination to play creatively round a theme. It is the triumph of positive logical principles, which in their nature can no longer be understood by purely formal psychology. Our meaning will be most clearly shown if we imagine the restraint imposed on us during thinking by a mathematical statement to be worked out. The direction of the thinking is in this case no longer subject to our desire. Of course our conversations do not deal with the acquisition of mathematical relations, but from the empirical arrangement of the things which affect the world of the child, touched on in the dialogues, there also proceeds an unavoidable compulsion to be treated and thought of in a definite way, whether, as botanical, zoological, or geographical objects they belong to nature or, as technical, historical, or social facts they belong to culture. As far as concerns the resultant positive logical tendencies which play their part in influencing the course of the child's conversation, we must refer to the analysis in the individual discussions. We are quite aware of the fact that in this connection we have only performed the preliminary work towards later more thorough investigations.

An extremely important and in many cases decisive influence on the course of the child's utterances is to be attributed to the totality of impulses which proceed from the adult as conversation-partner. In this place we may disregard the fact that among the coefficients determining the utterances of adults many still remain unknown.

We referred in the introduction to the lack of steadiness revealed occasionally in the graph of the child's mental development. We meet less of this in the conversations than might have been expected from the emphasis laid on this subject and the amount of space devoted to it. But it is easy to understand from the nature of these mental ruptures that they take place in secret. We get clear reflections of sudden changes mirrored in conversation 60 (ambition) and T's utterances quoted on pp. 235 f. (jealousy). Whereas emotions such as ambition and jealousy proceed from the adequate social conditions of the environment and to some degree attack the child unawares, yet he behaves spontaneously-creatively towards other situations and by this means suddenly advances himself one stage further in his development. We have been able to refer to several creative acts of this kind in the individual conversations.

4. Pedagogical Considerations

We stated in the introduction that almost all the conversations afford pedagogically a certain additional yield, although only a few conversations were carried on with a definitely pedagogical intention. As may be estimated from the results to be displayed here, they have at least this advantage over many other pedagogical investigations, that they were not thought out and constructed far removed from practice in the study, but possess the greatest degree of approximation to reality. Those people who have had the responsibility of training children and have moulded the innumerable collisions between theory and practice into an elastic educational front, will have little time for the advice of those pedagogues of the study who cling tightly to principles. What we attempt to give here is a piece of empirical pedagogy, small though it be, i.e. we reveal how instruction, information, and will formation towards certain goals is and can be realized.

At this point something ought to be said about the ideals of the home in which our children grew up, but the reader will understand the psychological restraint against such an undertaking and also will not really need such an explicit formulation of these ideals, for he will probably have been able to form an accurate idea of the home for himself from the conversations.

Empirical pedagogy! It does not overlook as easily as constructive pedagogy, the counter-effects which proceed from the child to the adult, counter-effects which with good reason may be claimed to be educational. In another place we have expressed our views in a somewhat more general way, about the shaping process still so neglected by science, to which parents are subjected in their intercourse with their children.[1] Here we may stress the fact that very

---

[1] Katz, *Erziehung*.

definite typical attitudes of the child induce correlative typical attitudes in the adult, which in course of time become habitual. The social psychology of marriage has not yet been written, and will have to deal with those qualities which are developed in the parents under the influence of the natural incompleteness of children which must be taken into account in their education. So far as moral qualities are concerned, the developed qualities are really all in the direction of passivity ; patience, calmness, self-control, devotion, self-renunciation, chivalry, and thoughtfulness might be mentioned. The countless questions put to us as parents set our didactive disposition in motion, and the child is, as we have seen above, a merciless questioner, who starts from the assumption that the parents know the answer to everything.

It will be found stated in some conversations that we have endeavoured to follow in the footsteps of Socrates in answering the children's questions, in so far as this method is adapted to young questioners. It has also been seen from the dialogues that the impetuous questions of the children sometimes could only be answered by a " you'll find that out when you're older ". We allowed ourselves to be led almost entirely by the children's need of enlightenment and endeavoured to keep indigestible mental fare away from them. It will perhaps be objected that the conversations seem to show that the children were informed about many unchildish subjects, which lay far beyond their mental horizon. Our reply to that objection is this. The children in a cultured family are in contact with many things which in an uncultured family remain hidden from them until they go to school or even later. During a conversation of adults at table the name Homer or Goethe is mentioned, and it would be false didactic purism not to reply to a child's question about it, that the one was a famous Greek and the other the greatest German poet. The child sees himself surrounded by reproductions of Dürer which he can thoroughly understand, and by etchings of Rembrandt, the content of which is clear to him. When he asks therefore about the people who made these works, ought he not to be told about the great masters in simple language ? At table foreign parts of the world are mentioned, where relatives live, and the natives of these places are discussed. Ought the child, whose imagination is aroused by this, to be told nothing of Africa and America, of negroes and Red Indians, if he wants to know about them ? During our conversations at table we endeavoured to prevent the children from hearing anything which might harm them, but the conversation could not be carried on so that it was composed only of matters which the children could understand. Most of it passes clean through the sieve of their interest without having had any perceptible effect, but some reappears much later, to the great astonishment of the parents, absolutely in the right place and properly understood, although at the time when it was received by the child's mentality it could scarcely have been understood. The amount of seed for later development, which can be stored up by a child living in a good intellectual atmosphere, can scarcely be estimated, and certainly cannot be estimated highly enough.

All pedagogues concerned with the will have emphasized the great importance for schooling the will of the formation of fixed habits which control the daily work. Amongst the accustomed habits developed by us we must mention the prayer which followed the evening talk, where strength for good conduct on the next day was to be collected. The talk is bound to the presence of a second person, but the prayer is not ; thus T. informed us that he had prayed by himself when the parents were away from home and he was alone in bed. We can be expected to furnish neither experimental proof nor enumerated examples of our statement that the talks, searching of conscience and evening prayer really had a very favourable influence, but it is our unshakeable conviction that this is so. We felt our educational task heightened immediately we introduced these methods. But even if we ourselves had not observed it, they would still have been justified because they gave to the children themselves the possibility of an abreaction and because they contributed towards shaping for the children a life freer from petty cares, which in reality seem petty only to the adult.

The close-knit nature of the ideology of the family, which meets the child as an educational force, usually suffers from the totally different attitude of the domestic staff. In various places in the conversations we had to speak about the educational counter-influence of the nursemaid as for instance when she ordered T. to keep his hands under the bedclothes, behaviour which had been expressly forbidden by the parents, so that T. had formed the opposite habit. In this case it is a question of only a single action, which of course cannot do any great damage to a habit already firmly implanted, but the situation is more serious with those influences which the child receives through tales of horror, and the not always harmless nursemaid's stories. In view of the child's receptivity towards such influences their effect is incalculable and is not so easily neutralized by counter-doses. In an uncontrolled hour the young child is suddenly attacked by things from which he has been carefully shielded. We were particularly sorry that in the field of religious education, where we were trying to put fixed principles into operation, the effect of the pedagogically untrained domestic staff could be observed. It is indeed almost a lucky accident—and this pessimistic view is based not merely on our own experience but on that of many other parents—to get a helper in the child's education, who falls in with the aims of the responsible authority so far as education, training and original pedagogical talent (the last the most important of the three) is concerned. In view of the prevailing conditions it was almost the lesser evil that the children saw through the weaknesses of the " aunts ", for by this means both they and their educational influence lost considerably in authority.

INDEX OF AUTHORS